NO SUGAR IN ME

Sugar is Out! Get Your Health Back!

A Note From The Author

In writing this book, I've had the opportunity to consult with fitness experts, medical experts, nutritionists, and others and these are my takes on what I learned from them.

Any changes to your dietary lifestyle should always be consulted with your doctor.

This book discusses sugar in its many forms.

When I reference natural sugar in the following pages, I'm referring to the sugar that naturally comes in the real food you're eating (like fruit). When I say processed, refined, or added sugar, I'm referring to the sugar that has been taken out of something natural, stripped of anything other than the sweetness and calories and put into other foods for taste. When discussing artificial sweeteners, I always refer to them as artificial.

Dedication

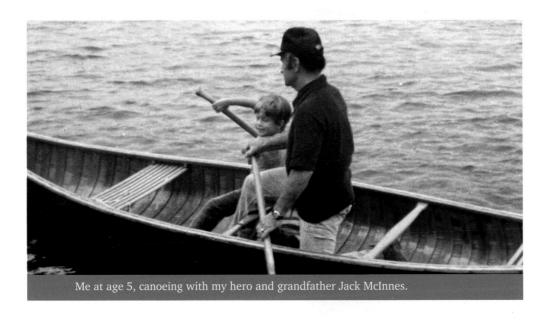

Me at age 5, canoeing with my hero and grandfather Jack McInnes.

To my grandfather, Jack McInnes, who taught me that no one can believe in yourself, as much as you.

To my parents, Margie and Rick, who instilled in me that all my dreams were possible, but you need to work hard to achieve them.

To my brother, Derek, who is the smartest entrepreneur I know, best brother someone could ask for, and who gave me my first opportunity to start my entrepreneurial journey.

To my daughters, Summer & Ivy, I hope to lead by example through hard work, persistence, and self-belief. I love you more than you will ever know.

To my wife, Mel, whose unconditional support, love, and selflessness is what I value the most. Thank you for being you.

Lastly, this book is dedicated to all of you who have struggled with eating, sugar consumption and achieving a healthy lifestyle. I truly understand where you are coming from as I've been there myself and hope this book helps show you that it's possible to improve by implementing even the smallest of changes. Believe me, you will never look back!

– Brad Woodgate

About The Author

Brad Woodgate is a self-made serial entrepreneur, who turned a thirty-thousand-dollar investment into over a billion dollars in sales. Having launched several successful companies over the past 21 years in the health and wellness space, he managed over 500 employees, launched over 700 products, and distributed to more than 50 countries. Through all of this, he learned what works in this space and what doesn't.

Over the years, Brad also helped many people and celebrities reach their wellness goals. In 2015, based on his own health concerns, Brad took a very strong interest in the effects of refined sugar on our health. This led to the establishment of the No Sugar Company in late 2018, which quickly grew and significantly disrupted the food industry globally.

Brad feels strongly that the No Sugar In Me™ lifestyle will be one of the biggest revolutions in the nutrition industry to date and has written this book to elevate the awareness as to why refined sugar is detrimental to our health and how to reduce or eliminate it from our daily diets.

Brad lives in Toronto, Canada, with his wife Mel and two girls, Summer and Ivy.

Table Of Contents

Introduction

HOW NO SUGAR IN ME CAME TO BE

Every kid should have a hero growing up. For me, my hero wasn't a caped crime fighter, a Hollywood action star, or a muscled-up jock. I was fortunate enough to be related to one. My hero was my grandfather, Jack McInnes, but it wasn't just a familial bond that made me look up to him. My grandfather won the Memorial Cup in hockey, became a professional hockey player drafted by the NHL's Boston Bruins, and competed in the British Empire Games in canoeing. He achieved all of these athletic accomplishments while standing only 5 foot 8 inches tall. To say he had to work extremely hard and be persistent in his goals would be an understatement. If that wasn't impressive enough, due to an injury, he left athletics, took interest in medicine and became one of the leading heart surgeons in the country. Now those are some big shoes to fill!

With the shadow of a pro athlete in my family history, it's no wonder I always wanted to be a professional athlete myself. It became my mission!

My sport of choice was basketball. I would wake up at 6AM every day and practice dribbling, spent hours each day perfecting my game and pushing myself to get better. In the end, I became a really decent player with moderate success at the college level, but for some reason I was just falling short of getting to the next level.

Health and fitness were always a part of my life. With a superhero grandfather like that, how could it not be? But, for someone who was so fitness oriented, spent so many hours being active, and took time to make food choices that I thought were in my best interests, I was always more or less chubby. To make matters even more frustrating, my brother, was a lean, mean, athletic

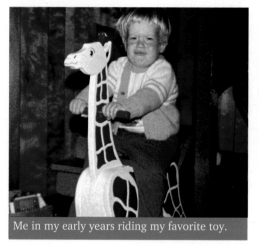
Me in my early years riding my favorite toy.

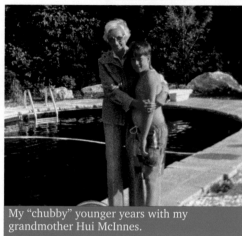
My "chubby" younger years with my grandmother Hui McInnes.

machine, without even paying attention to what he ate or trying as hard as I did. Sure, I wasn't obese, but you wouldn't exactly think 'athlete' when you saw me.

In spite of my efforts and true passion for sports, something was clearly holding me back from my full athletic potential.

What Was I Doing Wrong?

I left no stone unturned in trying to find the answer, testing out different diets, counting calories and had varied successes. But a true game changer came to me later in life by saying goodbye to processed sugar. Not only did I lose weight, but my energy spikes and crashes disappeared, my mood improved, and I felt and slept considerably better.

By now, it shouldn't surprise you that I didn't become a professional basketball player. But out of the ashes of that unrealized dream, something much, much bigger was born. At that time, not even I would have predicted that I'd be working with

celebrities on their diets, taking on the giants in the well-established food industry, breaking through the protocol of "how things are done" and actually achieving great successes. And yet, that is exactly what happened. For over 2 decades now, I've been credited as a "nutrition guru" by innovating products that are designed to help you achieve your health and fitness goals.

My grandfather used to say: "In persistency, lies victory." I wrote this book with the intention of empowering you to be persistent in your pursuit of health, share what I've learned about sugar and its detriment on our wellbeing and offer tools, guidance, and resources to hit your goals towards living your best life.

This book isn't an all-or-nothing detox or a quick-fix diet. It isn't a cookbook either. Instead, this book is about changing your lifestyle and is chockful of useful information about refined sugar and why some physicians consider it a legal and socially accepted toxin.[1]

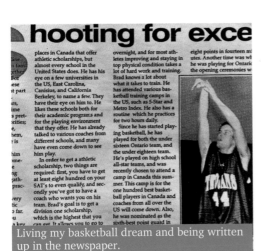

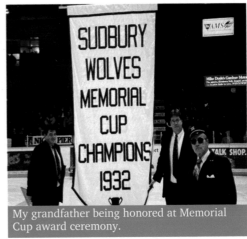

places in Canada that offer athletic scholarships, but almost every school in the United States does. He has his eye on a few universities in the US, East Carolina, Canisius, and California Berkeley, to name a few. They have their eye on him to. He likes these schools both for their academic programs and for the playing environment that they offer. He has already talked to various coaches from different schools, and many have even come down to see him play.

In order to get a athletic scholarship, two things are required: first, you have to get at least eight hundred on your SAT's to even qualify, and secondly you've got to have a coach who wants you on his team. Brad's goal is to get a division one scholarship, which is the highest that you can get. It allows you to go to

overnight, and for most athletes improving and staying in top physical condition takes a lot of hard work and training. Brad knows a lot about what it takes to train. He has attended various basketball training camps in the US, such as 5-Star and Metro Index. He also has a routine which he practices for two hours daily.

Since he has started playing basketball, he has played for both the under sixteen Ontario team, and the under eighteen team. He's played on high school all-star teams, and was recently chosen to attend a camp in Canada this summer. This camp is for the one hundred best basketball players in Canada and coaches from all over the US will come down. Also, he was nominated as the sixth-best point guard in

eight points in fourteen minutes. Another time was wl he was playing for Ontario the opening ceremonies w

Living my basketball dream and being written up in the newspaper.

My grandfather being honored at Memorial Cup award ceremony.

In Chapter 1, I'll share my personal journey of discovering the benefits of eliminating refined sugar, and how it led to an establishment of the No Sugar Company. In Chapter 2, different types of sugar will be discussed, how it became mass-produced and mass-consumed, and reveal a few unexpected sources of foods with high-sugar content. Following this, Chapter 3 will briefly review some clinical research linking this common ingredient to several serious health conditions and concerning trends globally. This is shared not to scare you but more so to elevate your awareness of the dangers of added sugars and motivate you to make a change in your life. In Chapter 4, I'll share my experiences and advice on how to reduce if not completely eliminate refined sugar from your diet.

Chapter 5 will bring some light to a very popular keto diet and tips on how to be successful while on it. In Chapter 6, I offer some practical advice that will help you prepare and substitute some common meals and snacks with healthier alternatives. My method will allow you to formulate your own approach to sugar and create a plan of mindful and intentional eating that works best for you. In Chapter 7, I will

speak about how to approach the topic of refined sugar with children. This topic is near and dear to my heart, as I am a proud father myself and can see immediate first-hand effects on how sugar highs and lows affect children's moods and behavior. Here, I will share some tips on what worked well in our home. In Chapter 8, we will address what our No Sugar Company is doing and our commitment to driving a change in this space. And lastly, we do end on a delicious note presenting you with a wide variety of elevated-cooking recipes that fit no-sugar diet as well as other diets like keto or plant-based. This tasty line up is sure to impress your pickest eaters and guests.

I hope that the story of my personal journey will inspire you to question your own relationship with refined sugar and perhaps, make a change as well. It doesn't have to be drastic or dramatic, but even the smallest of changes can make a big difference in the long run. The benefits of reducing your sugar intake can lead to better health outcomes, and that in and of itself is the best investment you can make.

Chapter 01

TAKING ON THE GIANTS

My personal struggles with weight, mood, and energy were an authentic motivator to understand my body and heal myself. Through research and efforts, I eventually managed to look and feel better, and am proud to say, even come close to rivaling my brother and his washboard abs. Out of all those efforts, an idea was born for a wellness initiative that led to a longstanding career in the nutritional industry.

When I was in my last year of University, my brother Derek and I launched a nutraceutical company called Wellnx Life Sciences (with plenty of help from Mom). Derek had worked in the industry for several years already, had his master's degree in nutrition and was working on completing his PhD. He had the knowledge, and I had the "never give up attitude." Our very first product was a weight management supplement called Diet Care.

To say that it wasn't an overnight success would be an understatement. For the first three years, like so many other startups, we struggled to stay afloat and cover our expenses. We didn't have a proven track record, established credibility, or connections in the industry. My role was to commercialize the product. I was told "NO" a lot. But I was hungry and determined, and personally interpreted every "NO" as a "maybe not right now." So, I kept showing up and the persistence paid off!

For the first seven years, I didn't take a single vacation and became relentless in trying to innovate and gain distribution in the biggest retailers in the world, including *Costco*,

Walmart, Target, Loblaws, Walgreens, Kroger, and many others. Our products worked and people started to take notice.

As our company began to garner attention, I was personally building a reputation and was frequently asked for advice on fitness and nutrition, eventually working with celebrities like Carmen Electra, Holly Madison, Tami Roman, and others.

In spite of our success in the weight loss and sports nutrition categories, I always felt there was a lot more impact to be made as there are millions of people who struggle with weight-loss but even more people who suffer from serious health conditions related to their nutrition. Instead of trying to address specific health conditions once they are already a problem, I wanted to focus on prevention. As I spent more time in the industry, learning about nutrition and common ingredients, I began to uncover the dangers of one commonly used ingredient on our overall health: processed sugar.

And quite quickly, I became obsessed with it.

The more I learned, the more it scared me. At that time, the no sugar idea was so novel and unappealing that even the name "NO SUGAR COMPANY" was unclaimed and untrademarked. I grabbed it and began my mission. This is truly where things blew up!

I had an inkling that it would be an uphill climb as nearly every large food manufacturer relies on refined sugar or some form

of it when creating their products. I wanted to do things differently. I wanted to create a line of products that don't rely on cheap, processed fillers devoid of nutritional value. My mission was to create a lifestyle and a movement centered around health without any compromises.

It took a lot of grit to go against the grain, learn about healthy alternatives, and zig when everyone is zagging. On more than one occasion, I was told "that's not how it's done" or "no one will pay premium for a product in this category." But out of big challenges come big rewards. We originally started with two products, No Sugar Keto Cups/Bombs and No Sugar Keto Bars, and, based on growing demand, are now thrilled to have expanded our product line into nut clusters, kid's snacks, cereal, snacking chocolate, coffee, and much more. All of which are made with the same premise of No Sugar: Great taste and high-quality, clean ingredients. Although our brand loyalists include those following the keto diet as well as diabetics, our customer base is really anyone who is interested in reducing their sugar intake (more on that in Chapter 8).

I am beyond excited to say that no sugar movement is rapidly growing and something that people are supporting in their choice of products they buy and consume and, more importantly, by making changes in their overall lifestyle. As a growing community, we are raising awareness of the importance of nutrition and avoidance of refined sugar in its mass-produced state.

Our mission at No Sugar Co. is to connect us not only through food, but also to create a safe place where we can support and learn from one another and have access to technology that will empower us to succeed. More on our tech efforts to come soon. For now, let me share the benefits you can expect to see once you adopt the No Sugar In Me lifestyle.

Benefits of No Sugar In Me

There is much to be gained by cutting out refined sugars, and here are a few key outcomes that you may see yourself.

Weight loss

You'll lose weight if you eliminate or reduce refined sugar, especially around your belly. [2] And for bonus points, bloating will fade away, too. Sugar is a natural

Clearer, younger looking skin

Cutting out processed sugars will also lead to visible results in your skin as well. Eating too much sugar can cause inflammation. Inflammation can lead to flare ups and aggravate conditions such as acne and eczema and also cause breakdown of collagen fibers, which accelerates aging. [3] Thus, saying no to sugar can make us not only feel good on the inside, but also make us look our best on the outside.

Increased energy

If you thought a sugar rush was a way to get an energy boost and get you through that afternoon slump, going sugar-free is actually a much better way to avoid those energy dips to begin with. In fact, sugar crashes and greater fatigue often follow

> ## "Saying no to sugar is the best way to have consistent power in your tank throughout the day versus inconsistent ups and downs."

appetite inducer, meaning that the sweeter the foods that we eat are, the more we will crave them. This cycle often leads to overconsumption of empty calories and overeating. Stopping that cycle by cutting out refined sugar will help us achieve and maintain healthy weight.

consumption of sugary snacks or drinks.[4] So saying no to sugar is the best way to have consistent power in your tank throughout the day versus inconsistent ups and downs.

Better sleep

Interrupted slumber is out. Deeper sleep is in. When our blood sugars are in balance, our hormones allow us to establish healthier sleep patterns including staying asleep with fewer interruptions.[5]Dr Michael Breus, who specializes in sleep disorders, explains that "too much sugar leads to a tendency to eat later in the day...[t]hat adversely affects sleep, and your disrupted sleep will, in turn, produce an even greater craving for sugar the next day. The vicious circle is complete."[6]So kick the sugar habit and you'll be more likely to get a good night's rest.

Better Focus

That foggy feeling will be gone when you drop added sugar from your life. Tests have shown that individuals who regularly overconsume high levels of sugar have significantly lower cognitive performance in verbal and visual memory.[7]With the stress that sugar puts on your brain gone, you'll be thinking clearer and accomplishing more throughout the day.

Better smile

Whiter, healthier teeth await you. Your overall oral health will see a huge improvement. Why? Sugar is one of the favorite food sources not only for us, but also for the bacteria in our mouths! As the bacteria thrives on sugar, this will increase our chances for tooth decay, cavities, chronic inflammation, and gum disease. Reducing sugar intake would decrease your likelihood of these oral complications.[8]So protect your pearly whites by cutting out processed sugar.

Increased Performance When Active

By having more consistent energy levels through the day, you'll want to hit the gym, be more active, and experience greater impact from those efforts.

Plus, you'll have a much greater health outlook for the rest of your life: Cutting out refined sugar decreases risks of having serious health conditions such as obesity, diabetes, heart disease, high cholesterol, liver disease, chronic inflammation, and more. Also, you can expect to see an improvement in your mood as well. It seems that anxiety loves added sugars, especially during sugar crashes when we are most likely to feel irritable, worried or sad.[9]So keeping refined sugar out of our lives will help us regulate not only energy levels but also positive emotions.

The key reason why I decided to write this book is in hopes of elevating this topic and to help establish healthier habits for ourselves and our future generations. Chances are that if you're reading this, you already have some level of concern when it comes to this ingredient.

So, let's get started!

Chapter 02

UNCOVERING THE BITTER TRUTH ABOUT SUGAR

First off, not all sugar is the same. In this section, I'll explain the different types of sugar, review its usage over time and how it evolved, and offer scientific evidence on its detrimental impact on our health and why some experts refer to it as modern day "toxin." [10]

Not all Sugar Is Created Equal

When you really want to define sugar, you have to look at it as one of two things: Natural Sugar and Refined Sugar (or processed and added sugar to be more precise). The differences are quite obvious, but the lines of distinction have been intentionally blurred by the food industry to trick you into buying products that are not honestly presented. Let's cut through the noise and clearly define the two.

Natural Sugars

Naturally occurring sugar is the one that appears in whole foods such as fruit, vegetables, dairy, and whole grains, which contain nutrients that support our overall health. Because the sugar found in whole foods is combined with fiber, vitamins, and minerals needed by our bodies, I would consider this as an essential part of our diet. Simply put, this sugar isn't the enemy.

Refined Sugars

It is refined, processed sugar that's devoid of any nutritional value that causes issues. Some have told me "Brad, sugar is sugar, and our bodies process it in the exact same way," which is true. Sugar in any form produces blood sugar and insulin spikes. However, we typically wouldn't eat an entire basket of strawberries in one sitting because of all the extra fiber that they contain, which fills us up. This stops us from overeating. On the other hand, it isn't unheard of to eat a whole candy bar at a time, simply because they don't lead to satiety in the same way. In other words, what makes a big difference in this case is the total package of the "good stuff" that whole foods sugars are combined with, versus refined sugars that we artificially infuse our foods with.

Acceptable sugar comes in food naturally. The sugar you don't need is the granulated sugar on your kitchen counter that's been added to the packaged foods you buy at the grocery store.

You may also be wondering where honey and maple syrup fit into the sugar equation. Both are fair options to be used in baking and as pour-over sweeteners, but they, too, undergo a refinement process like table sugar that strips away much (and in some cases all) of their vital nutrients.

Artificial Sweeteners
Artificial Sweeteners are synthetic sugar substitutes, which are more concentrated and intensely sweeter than natural sugars. In some cases, they can be more than 13,000 times sweeter than natural sugars! Artificial sweeteners differ from one another in how they are derived, their intensity of sweetness, but most importantly in how they affect our bodies. The most commonly used artificial sweeteners approved by the Food and Drug Administration (FDA) include: Acesulfame, aspartame, sucralose,

neotame, and saccharin, many of which come with a warning label. While the FDA has cleared these sweeteners for public use, they do recognize the potential for some harm since research has found data that may link them to negative health effects, although not conclusive in their opinion. Here is a brief glimpse into each of these sweeteners.

Acesulfame is an artificial sweetener that has a checkered past that has linked it to a host of negative side effects, including the disruption of metabolic processes, appetite interference and irregularities, weight gain, and blood sugar spikes. It is about 200 times sweeter than sugar.

Aspartame, which is 200 times sweeter than sugar, took 16 years to gain FDA approval. It is found in many leading brands but is accompanied by an FDA warning label on the box. Research has linked it to cancer, seizures, headaches, ADHD, depression, dizziness, weight gain, and birth defects.

Sucralose may be one of the most common of the artificial sweeteners, but it isn't without its own questionable health concerns. Linked to increased weight gain, fat storage, and a greater appetite, it frequently does the opposite of what you'd want from a zero-calorie sweetener in that it makes you want to eat more food. Being 600 times sweeter than sugar, sucralose packs a sweet punch that could also damage intestinal flora, impacting your metabolism and immune system.

Neotame is a whopping 7,000 to 13,000 times sweeter than sugar and has been linked to causing abdominal pain in those that ingest it. In a more concerning note, research indicates that it can cause brain damage in the fetus.

Saccharin is up to 700 times sweeter than regular sugar and has been linked to causing headaches and diarrhea. The FDA had a warning label on this artificial sweetener from 1997 to 2001. It didn't suddenly become safe though. The National Toxicology Program Board of Scientific Counselors concluded that saccharin should still be considered a cancer-causing chemical, in spite of the US Congress removing the warning label.

Given all the findings mentioned above and the elevated health risks they are associated with, my opinion is that those artificial sweeteners should be avoided.[11]

Erythritol and Stevia
In addition to the aforementioned artifi-cial sweeteners, the FDA and many other international governing bodies have also approved Erythritol and Stevia as a natural sugar substitute.

Erythritol and Stevia, are naturally occurring sugar substitutes derived from plants and receive their sweetness from plant leaves. Stevia is extracted from the leaves of a plant in the sunflower family called Stevia Rebaudiana. Erythritol is also found naturally in some foods like grapes, pears, peaches, mushrooms, and watermelon. Both are natural sugar substitutes that taste great and, most importantly, both are considered safe.[12]

In order to meet the regulation requirements of the FDA, Stevia needs to go through a filtering process to achieve purity and the right concentration. It is available suspended in liquid, granulated, or powdered form and is 300 times sweeter than sugar.[13] Erythritol on the other hand is milder, as it is estimated to be 70% as sweet as sugar.[14]

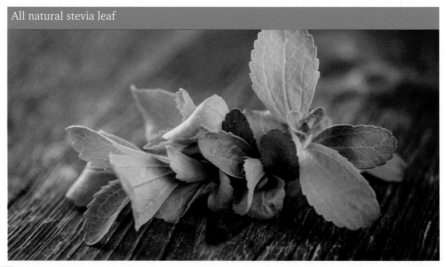
All natural stevia leaf

Erythritol and Stevia can help stabilize blood sugar levels by slowing down gastric emptying and the release of sugar into your bloodstream. As a result, you will stay full longer, reducing your appetite and cravings in the process. It is also considered safe for those at risk or diagnosed with diabetes, or those adhering to a keto diet as it does not change blood sugar, glucose, insulin levels, cholesterol, or triglycerides. [15]

While both Stevia and Erythritol are considerably more expensive than other sweeteners and refined sugar, most of the time, you do need only a small quantity because of their sweetness levels. In my opinion, if you are going to use a sugar substitute, Erythritol and Stevia are your very best options.

The Many Names of Sugar That Can Confuse You

It should be pretty easy and obvious to know if something you're buying at your local grocery store has processed sugar in it, right? Wrong. Sugar has many names and many forms. Food manufacturers have gotten a lot smarter over the years in hiding the sugars through its many names.

There are currently 72 different names for sugar and it's very probable that this list will continue to evolve. [16]

- Agave nectar
- Barbados sugar
- Barley malt
- Barley malt syrup
- Beet sugar
- Blackstrap molasses
- Brown rice syrup
- Brown sugar
- Buttered syrup
- Cane juice
- Cane juice crystals
- Cane sugar
- Caramel
- Carob syrup
- Castor sugar
- Coconut palm sugar
- Coconut sugar
- Confectioner's sugar
- Corn sweetener
- Corn syrup
- Corn syrup solids
- Crystal line fructose
- Date sugar
- Dehydrated cane juice
- Demerara sugar
- Dextrin
- Dextrose
- Diastatic malt
- Diatase
- Ethyl Maltol
- Evaporated cane juice
- Free-flowing brown sugars
- Fructose
- Fruit juice
- Fruit juice concentrate
- Galactose
- Glucose
- Glucose solids
- Golden sugar
- Golden syrup
- Grape sugar
- HFCS (High-Fructose Corn Syrup)
- Honey
- Icing sugar
- Invert sugar
- Lactose
- Malt syrup
- Maltodextrin
- Maltol
- Maltose
- Mannose
- Maple syrup
- Molasses
- Muscovado
- Oat syrup
- Palm sugar
- Panocha
- Panela
- Powdered sugar
- Raw sugar
- Refiner's syrup
- Rice syrup
- Saccharose
- Sorghum Syrup
- Sucrose
- Sugar (granulated)
- Sweet Sorghum
- Syrup
- Treacle
- Tapioca syrup
- Turbinado sugar
- Yellow sugar

The Proliferation of Refined Sugar

How did sugar become such an integral part of our Western diet? Here is a brief story of this mighty sweet ingredient that was once considered a rarity and has now become nearly impossible to escape.

The earliest records show that over 8,000 years ago, humans in New Guinea discovered plants that had sweetness and chewed on the reeds to extract it.[17] Its existence was relatively insignificant until the discovery in India was made on how to transform sugarcane juice into crystallized form. This was a true game changer in the story of sugar, as it became significantly easier to store, cook with, and transport.

From there, sugar was used for a wide range of medicinal purposes, being prescribed for everything from fever, cough, pectoral ailments, painful bladder and kidney issues, chapped lips and stomach diseases.[18] Even today, in some parts of the word where antibiotics aren't easily accessible or aren't effective, sugar is still being used for treatment of wounds. Sugar granules act as a natural antibiotic of sorts, as they absorb the moisture on a wound and prevent harmful bacteria from forming, thus minimizing infection, and expediting the healing process.[19]

Aside from medicinal use, once sugar made its way around the world to Europe, it became a symbol for royalty where it was considered so valuable that in some cases, this "sweet salt" was locked up in sugar safes.[20]

Up until 150 years ago, aside from royalty, average people only consumed sugar by eating natural foods. Like many other commodities, sugar became accessible for

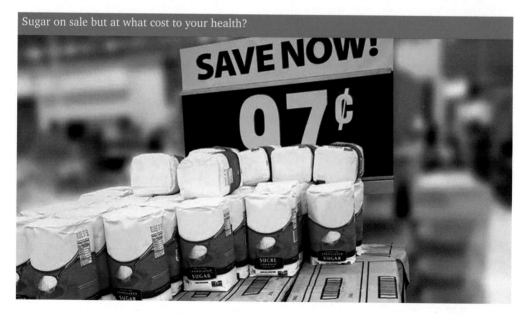

Sugar on sale but at what cost to your health?

the masses in the late 18th century, when technology enabled us to refine sugar and its many derivatives on a large scale. And now, in today's society, I would argue that sugar in its mass-produced state has evolved into a symbol for overindulgence and is no better than cigarette smoking.

The obsession with refined sugar and its many forms has grown exponentially worldwide. As our consumption of sugar keeps increasing, its costs are actually going down, getting cheaper and cheaper over time. It is projected that the cost of sugar will decrease from 17 cents to 14 cents US per pound in the span of a decade.[21] The unfortunate implication of such decrease in cost is that refined sugar is expected to become even more accessible and eaten in the future.

Maybe governments will eventually step in like they did with the tobacco industry but until then, the damage to the health of humankind will continue to proliferate.

Why is sugar so popular? Well, for one, sugar is a dream ingredient for mass-produced products for most large food manufacturers. It is a relatively inexpensive ingredient that tastes good and also increases food shelf life.[22] Additionally, sugar stimulates our appetite, driving you to eat more. It is no wonder that the food industry invests billions of dollars in food engineering to ensure that sugar levels are optimal for just that perfect pop of "bet you can't eat just one bite" addiction and billions more in marketing to extend their reach.

The Food Industry's Dirty Little Secret: SUGAR IS EVERYWHERE

Many of us can hum along with the words from the famous Mary Poppins song: "A spoon full of sugar makes the medicine go down" Well, gleeful as that may be, it is one of the many indicators that sugar has made its way into popular culture and our diets. Refined sugar is prevalent not only in obvious sweet items like chocolate bars, gummies, pastries, and soda but also in many savory items and even in medications and vitamins.

It is included in most leading brands of:
- Barbeque, pizza and pasta sauces
- Ketchups
- Salad dressings
- Cereals
- Packaged canned fruit
- Granola bars
- Crackers, soups
- Breads, bagels, pastries
- French fries
- Dried fruit
- Jerky and other cured meat
- Instant / flavored oatmeal
- Yogurts
- Sports / energy drinks and flavored waters
- Specialty coffees
- Sticky rice used for sushi
- Many leading cough syrups and chewable multivitamins

In addition to calling sugar derivatives by its many names, food manufacturers often combine different types of sugar to ensure that refined sugar doesn't appear as the top ingredient on the food label. This is just another trick up their sleeve, which allows them to increase the amount of sugar they pump our food with. Just take a look at any nutrition label in your local grocery store and you'll see a number of examples of hidden sugars that have been added to your food.

The last thing to note is that "low-fat" and "fat-free" foods are usually amongst the worst offenders when it comes to high sugar content. As food manufacturers extract natural fats from foods, the food itself loses a lot of flavor. As a result, refined sugar is often added to enhance the flavor profile.[23] You may ask, "So what, Brad, if the food tastes better with sugar, where is the harm in that?"

The unfortunate truth is that while our access and consumption of sugar exponentially increased, our bodies simply didn't evolve to keep up and process it in such high quantities.

That discrepancy between the quantities we are eating and our inability to properly digest it is causing an onslaught of health problems worldwide.

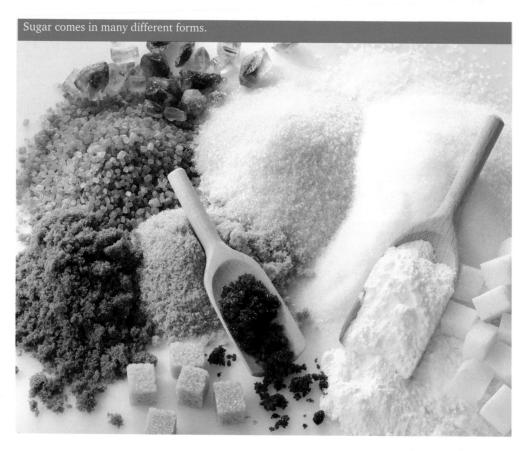

Sugar comes in many different forms.

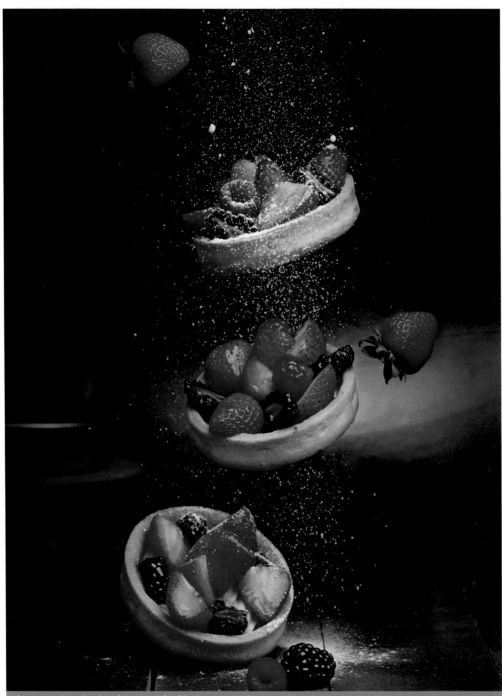

There are hundreds of grams of added sugar in desserts like these.

Chapter 03

SUGAR'S EROSION OF OUR HEALTH

I find it ironic that sugar was once used as medicine and is now considered by some as a toxin endangering our health. The unfortunate part is that it is easily accessible and its effects on our health are still being debated. Dr. Robert Lustig, a San Francisco-based endocrinologist argues: "This is a public health crisis. And when it's a public health crisis, you have to do big things and you have to do them across the board. Tobacco and alcohol are perfect examples. We have made a conscious choice that we're not going to get rid of them, but we are going to limit their consumption. I think sugar belongs in this exact same wastebasket." [24]

The fact is many of us are now eating foods that contain added sugars in nearly every meal. According to the World Health Organization, we should not be consuming more than 10 percent of our daily calories from sugar. And yet, more than 75 percent of Americans eat 2-3 times more than the recommended amount.[25] That adds up to 150lbs of sugar per year for an average person![26]

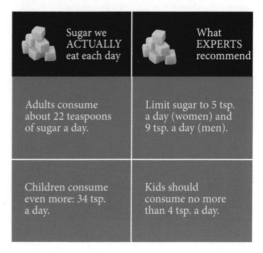

Sugar we ACTUALLY eat each day	What EXPERTS recommend
Adults consume about 22 teaspoons of sugar a day.	Limit sugar to 5 tsp. a day (women) and 9 tsp. a day (men).
Children consume even more: 34 tsp. a day.	Kids should consume no more than 4 tsp. a day.

Given that our metabolism and digestion systems have not evolved to process much more than the sugar found in two medium sized fruits per day, this elevated level of consumption puts our bodies at incredible risks, increasing our likelihood of all kinds of health complications. A growing number of medical and clinical studies are identifying sugar as the culprit, linking it to a heightened risk for weight gain, obesity, diabetes, heart disease, autoimmune conditions, chronic inflammation, brain conditions, liver disease, and premature aging. To keep things concise, in the next section, we will take a quick glance at four areas: fat, obesity, diabetes, and heart health in their relation to sugar. Entire books have been written on these topics, so I don't want to overwhelm you with the stats and clinical research. Having said that, if you are interested in learning more than what I've provided in this section, skip to Appendix C where I offer further information on how sugar has been linked to conditions referenced above along with corresponding research.

Fat and Sugar

It was in the mid-1950s when medical professionals started taking notice of increasing rates of obesity, diabetes, and heart disease. This triggered the debate of the dangers of Fat versus Sugar, with researchers divided into two polarizing camps. After much debate, fat was identified as the main culprit endangering humankind.

Decades later, something surprising was discovered: Three Harvard scientists who researched the dangers of fat vs. sugar and published a very influential study were actually paid by the sugar industry. Their findings concluded that sugar was a dental concern and instead told the public to be more concerned with fat.[27] According to the documentation that emerged since then, *The New York Times* reported that the payment equivalent in today's value of $50,000 US dollars was made by the Sugar Association to the three scientists that published the paper.[28] "This is quite what we had in mind and look forward to its appearance in print" read a message from the Sugar Association to one of the researchers.[29]

And yet, this type of biased research changed the perception that the world had of sugar and fat, along with the type of food that was produced and eaten. We were told to consider fat-free options for better health and not pay attention to sugar content. Sugar remained under the radar and was promoted as an energy-inducing, natural ingredient, intentionally blurring the important distinction between natural and refined sugars.

When the food manufacturers took out the fat, they were left with flavorless food and subsequently upped the sugar levels so consumers would find their products pleasant to eat. And in spite of us adhering to the recommendations made by the governing bodies and eating low-fat foods, heart disease, diabetes, and obesity rates continued to skyrocket.

Thus, as an aspiring athlete growing up in these times, I myself fell into the low-fat trap. I was told to lose weight and assumed that the fat intake was the problem, so I cut it out of my diet as much as possible. I even made efforts to limit carbs. What was left? Sugar! And I had a lot of sugar in my diet because I assumed it was necessary for energy and sustaining my high-intensity workouts. So as hard as tried, my efforts were futile, as the excess weight was slowly packing on. That is, until I changed my ways.

Some of you may ask if sugar was really the culprit for my weight gain. Fortunately for us, researchers all over the world are now raising the alarm bells on refined sugar. Sugar lobbyists are still hard at work, but their job is becoming exponentially harder as the science continues to explore the topic and, anecdotally, people like myself are seeing a difference in their own bodies once refined sugar is cut out.

Obesity and Sugar
It is no wonder that as our sugar consumption grew, our collective waistlines did as well. While sugar may not be identified yet as a direct cause of obesity or excessive weight gain, there is irrefutable evidence showing that the more sugar you eat, the higher your risk of being overweight and obese.[30]

Obesity, a condition associated with having too much body fat is on a rapid rise worldwide. According to the World Health Organization, obesity around the world has nearly tripled since 1975. Today, nearly 75 percent of American adults are classified as overweight as well as nearly 30 percent of children. On average, one out of three Americans is obese.[31]

Sadly, an obese person's risk of a heart attack is 3 times greater.[32] They are also 80 times more likely to develop Type 2 Diabetes compared to someone who has a healthy weight.[33]

Financially, obesity is also extremely expensive. Some estimates show that equivalent to nearly 10% of the US Gross Domestic Product is related to excessive weight gain, obesity, and indirect costs due to loss of productivity.[34]

Surprisingly, more than half of the world's population live in countries where more people die from being overweight than being underweight. That means overeating, a choice and condition that is preventable, is killing more people than starvation.

In 2016, almost 2 billion adults were considered overweight and more than a quarter of those were clinically obese.[35]

One thing that gained medical consensus is that the best way that an individual can treat or prevent obesity is to eat a healthy diet rich in whole foods and healthy fats, and low sugar.

On a more collective scale, governments, communities, policy makers, and food manufacturers need to offer proper education, support and foods in order to reverse this trend.

Diabetes and Sugar

Diabetes is a terrible disease with a high and rising prevalence worldwide. I have friends who suffer with the disease, so it hits close to home for me. There are two types of diabetes: Type 1, which happens due to immune system issues, and Type 2 that is mostly caused by diet. While the clinical community is still exploring the role of sugar in diabetes, it should be noted that sugar isn't currently marked as a direct cause, but more so as a correlation. In other words, science has proven that having a diet rich in sugar does make diabetes more likely.[36]

Between 1990 and 2010, the number of people with diabetes in the United States tripled.[37] As bleak as that sounds, there is incredibly encouraging insight that indicates a reduction in your body weight by even a small amount, such as 5 to 10 percent of your body weight, can lower your risk of developing metabolic conditions such as type 2 diabetes by 58 percent.[38] In other words, if you are 185 pounds and prediabetic, losing just 9 to 18 pounds can slash your chance of having diabetes by more than half. Take that and consider it all the more reason to say no to sugar.

Heart Health and Sugar

Your heart is far from immune from the damage caused by a diet high in added sugar. In a study published in 2014 in *JAMA Internal Medicine*, researchers discovered a link between a high- sugar diet and a greater risk of dying from heart disease. The 15-year study found that people who get 17% to 21% of their calories from added sugar had a 38% greater risk of dying from cardiovascular disease. They concluded that the more sugar a person's diet has, the higher the risk for heart disease and compromised cardiovascular health.[39]

In addition to that, in the case of diets that are rich in sugar, high blood pressure and a significant increase of chronic inflammation is seen. All of that means that you'll be on the fast track to heart disease.[40]

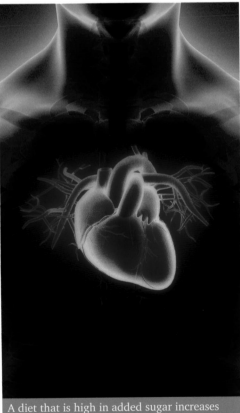

A diet that is high in added sugar increases your risk of death from heart disease.

Chapter 04

NO SUGAR, I AM SWEET ENOUGH!

With our No Sugar, I am Sweet Enough™ slogan, I wanted to highlight that it's important to have confidence within you, and have a reminder that you are sweet, strong, and amazing, which will only grow as you make positive choices for yourself. I know the No Sugar In Me lifestyle will work for anyone. I also know that most people should make the switch because refined sugar has long term effects on their health —often without them even knowing it until it becomes difficult to treat. Whenever I'm asked if no sugar will work, I ask those same people to answer a few questions about the role of sugar in their life. This is the perfect time for you to play along as well.

Below is a list of 20 questions. While reading them, count how many of these questions you answered 'Yes' to. The results will answer the following vital question about you, and only you: Do you have a problem with added sugar?

Pop Quiz: Do you Need Sugar in Your Life?
Do you crave sugar?
Do you need a sweet treat after a meal?
Do you find fruit 'not sweet enough' for you?
Are you hungry almost all the time?
Have you recently gained weight?
Do you find it nearly impossible to lose weight?
Do you struggle with bloating?
Do you experience mood swings?
Do you feel weak?
Have you recently lost muscle?
Have you lost the desire to workout?
Do you have joint pain?
Do you have little to no energy?

Do you have high blood pressure?
Do you frequently have an upset stomach?
Do you experience interrupted sleep?
Are you frequently confused or caught
off guard?
Is your skin prematurely wrinkled?
Do you have mouth pain and/or more cavities
than ever?
Are you experiencing break outs or acne?

How did you do? Did you answer 'Yes' to
more than 10 of these questions? More
than 15? All 20? The reality is that we will
all answer yes to some of these occasionally, but if you answered 'Yes' to more than
5 of these questions on any given day, it
may be indicative of a sugar dependency.
If that is the case, don't fret! This is the
perfect opportunity to make a change! It's
also a clear sign that you need to switch
to a No Sugar In Me lifestyle and join this
growing movement. Let's dive deeper into
what you can expect to gain by eliminating processed sugar from your life.

No Sugar In Me Lifestyle Questions
Some proponents of the no sugar movement argue that detoxes are necessary.
Others argue that all sugars including
that found in fruit, vegetables, and dairy
should be strictly avoided in order to
readjust our blood sugar levels as well
as our tastebuds. I believe in a more
moderate approach. Being aware of the
volume of sugar consumed and just as
importantly, the actual source of these
sugar matters.
Thus, my personal take is that not all
sugar is bad. It's the added, processed

sugar we need to stay away from. To help
provide more clarity on how I see the no
sugar lifestyle, here are the top 5 questions
I get asked the most often, along with
my answers.

1. *Can I eat fruit on a no sugar diet?* This
is my favorite question about the no sugar
lifestyle. My take on it is: Of course you
can eat it. In fact, you should eat fruit!
The answer is inextricably linked to the
nutritional profile of whole foods. Fruit is
packed with goodness that you need in the
form of nutrients, vitamins, and fiber. This
is the acceptable kind of sugar your body
can get. "If you eliminate fruits from your
daily diet you will be missing out on so
many benefits."

I should offer a brief caveat. By "fruit," I
mean literal fruit. I don't mean fruit drinks,
the added fruit that comes in some sugary
yogurts, "fruit flavored" ingredient claims
or dried fruits at the store, all of which
can be secretly packed with added sugars.
Avoid these missteps. Your brain will try
to rationalize with you and tell you it's still
"fruit." But it is not. Stick to the real, whole
foods and you'll be much better off.

If you can center your fruit intake around
lemons, limes, raspberries, strawberries,
blackberries, kiwis, grapefruit, avocado,
watermelon, cantaloupe, and peaches,
you'll be doing just fine. These fruits will
have the lowest impact on your overall
blood sugar levels, in addition to rejuvenat-
ing your body with healthy nutrients, vitamins, and minerals. Over time, your taste

buds will change so that you'll crave these great fruits. Eventually, the taste of dried fruits with added sugar will shock your tastebuds and you may surprise yourself and not enjoy them as much.

2. *If I quit added, processed sugars, will I lose my energy?* It's true that you might initially experience some fatigue in the early days of your No Sugar In Me lifestyle. Specifically, days 2 through 4 tend to be the toughest. But this won't last. By day 6, you are likely going to feel renewed, steady energy levels throughout the day. In fact, in the long run, a no sugar lifestyle will help you avoid the highs and lows of sugar cravings and their associated crashes. People who stick with the elimination of refined sugar will experience consistent levels of energy and mental clarity, which is a fantastic combination for optimal productivity.

3. *Will a no sugar lifestyle affect my workouts?* While it's true that muscle growth requires energy, and energy comes in large part from glucose, it's definitely a myth that going on the no added, processed sugar lifestyle will prevent you from building muscle. In fact, your body will do better at muscle growth once you switch to a diet rich in whole foods and their associated nutrient-rich forms of carbs, proteins, and fats.

4. *I am always on the go, how do I make No Sugar an option away from home?* Clearly, it's healthier if we cook at home and know what ingredients go into our meals, but you can absolutely eat at restaurants or cook in

batches and bring your Tupperware along. The important thing to remember when eating at a restaurant or at home is that you make an attempt to choose the healthier options. Plan ahead. If you have time, check out the menu before you arrive. Generally speaking, grilled, baked, or steamed options are always better than fried. When it comes to minimizing added sugars, try to avoid appetizers with heavy sauces, glazes, sugary drinks, and the dessert menu and you'll enjoy a dinner out without derailing your no sugar lifestyle for the day.

5. *Can I eat desserts or treats?* In short, yes. In my opinion, most diets fail long-term because they're too restrictive. So, if you want to live a lifestyle that's both healthy and realistic, you'll have to acknowledge that there's a middle path between gorging on added sugar and absolute sugar abstinence. I am also here to tell you that there are a growing list of responsible no or low sugar companies with great options for when that craving strikes.

6. *What should my kids eat?* It can be tough to get your kids on board with change, especially because so many foods are targeted directly at children with ambiguous terms like artificial sugar alcohols in the nutrition and likely untrue promises on the label. Look for the sugar content on any food you give your kids because even something as simple as a bowl of cereal may go beyond the daily recommended about of sugar they should be eating!
Now that we've addressed some of the most commonly asked questions about the

No Sugar In Me lifestyle, you're probably warming up to the idea of the change more than you ever anticipated. That's awesome! So now, ask yourself two critical questions:

What is your current relationship with refined sugar?

What do you want your relationship with refined sugar to be?

Define your no sugar goals and write them down. Why does a no sugar lifestyle matter to you? Do you want to reduce it or eliminate it? Do you want that change to be gradual or instant? Writing down your personal motivation for adopting this lifestyle and defining the goals you want to accomplish positions you for a higher likelihood of success.

Based on how you answer these questions, work your way through our suggestions outlined below. You may decide to reduce added sugars gradually or quit straight away. I've given you options and suggestions on how to work through both. These suggestions don't need to be done all at once, but each of them can help you on your path to succeeding with this life change.

While I personally decided to quit all refined sugars straight away and pushed through it allowing myself occasional cheat days, you may choose to reduce your sugar intake by a certain percentage or even work through the plan gradually.

As an added bonus, I included a 5-step Crush Your Sugar Craving™ tool below to help you overcome those moments when you're really craving that something sweet. You decide what works best for you and then apply the recommended steps accordingly.

How to Crush Your Sugar Cravings

Let's face it: Sugar cravings happen to all of us, very often, and sometimes several times throughout the day. What should we do in those moments of weakness? Crush that sugar craving is what we should do! Below is a tried and tested approach that I've developed for myself, friends, family, and customers, which will soon be more robust and available for free in our App. My method includes 5 simple steps and a bit of patience as you move through them. Note that timing is important: Spending at least 5 minutes for each step is critical in allowing that craving to subside. Let's walk through it together. Let's say that you're craving something sweet (insert your craving of choice here).

Step 1: Drink a glass of water.
Wait for 5 minutes. Note: Sometimes mindless eating is actually driven by thirst, so water is always a great place to start. Still craving it? Move to the next step.

Step 2: Distract yourself with a 5-minute activity.
Listen to your favorite song and dance. Think of something simple that forces your mind off your craving. Send someone a

text to tell them how much they mean to you. Watch a funny video. Read an article and learn something new. Note: We often eat out of boredom, so finding an activity to distract our focus can often redirect our attention and reduce our desire to eat. Still craving it? If yes, move to the next step.

Step 3: Grab a No Sugar substitute.

This is where planning ahead is key. You should have a well-stocked snack drawer in your pantry and fridge for moments like these. Naturally, I'd suggest any of our No Sugar Co. products at thenosugarcompany.com, after all, I want to be a part of the solution, along with other snacks like unsweetened popcorn, nuts, seeds, nut butters, cheese, pre-cut fresh fruit or vegetables, and dips like hummus. Ensure that your snacks are set to individual portions to avoid the temptation of overeating. If you're leaving home, make sure that you also have some of these snacks in your purse or car. Eat your no sugar snack mindfully by sitting down and wait for 5 minutes. Still craving that sugary snack? If yes, move to the next step.

Step 4: Brush Your Teeth or Chew Sugar-Free Gum.

Sounds simple, right? The feeling of clean teeth may be enough to deter you from eating again so go ahead and brush. An alternative to brushing your teeth is to use mouthwash. If you don't want to brush or rinse, go ahead and get a stick of sugar-free gum. As an added bonus, some say that chewing gum also acts as a way of toning facial muscles, sends a signal to your brain that you're already eating, and helps burn a small number of calories. Either way, it's a win-win, and this is definitely where I find most of my cravings stop. So, go ahead and chew for at least 5 minutes (or for some bonus points, even longer). Either way, your mouth will feel clean and refreshed and knowing that the snack will taste different after that minty flavor should be a great deterrent. Wait for 5 minutes and see how you feel. Still craving that sugary snack? If yes, move to the next step.

Step 5: Move Your Body.

There is nothing quite like physical activity to reset your body, mind, and even your cravings. It doesn't have to be anything too intense or time-consuming. In fact, just going for a quick walk or jog could do the trick. The point is to be moving your body for at least five minutes. This moves your mind away from the craving and onto something more proactive. Still craving that sugary snack? If yes, it's ok.

Final Deed: Take the item you were craving and eat it mindfully.

Eating shouldn't be associated with guilt. If you are still craving the item after going through all 5 steps above, sit down and eat it slowly. Enjoy it without distractions and truly taste the food. And if you got to this step, that's ok. You'll crush that sugar craving next time!

Do your best to document the frequency of your cravings and how successful you were in crushing them using this 5-step approach. Over time, you will notice that you're experiencing these cravings less frequently and crushing them more successfully. This is also where our No Sugar In Me app will become very useful, allowing you to track those cravings and crush them as they come! I am beyond excited that very soon, I will be able to offer the No Sugar In Me app for free to all of you! So follow us on social @nosugarcompany to grab your free No Sugar In Me app and use it as soon as it's available.

Getting to No Sugar In Me Gradually

Through my years of working to disrupt the food industry I've met a lot of experts in the realm of weight loss, fitness, health, and wellness. I've tried to understand our ability to make significant, positive change to our health by speaking with dietitians, personal trainers, medical doctors, psychologists, life coaches, and just regular people struggling to understand their health and make a change. While there's a lot to unpack from all sides, I've distilled their greatest advice into these 10 easy steps you can make to see positive change in your life.

1. Eat Frequently, Mindfully and Never Starve Yourself: It may seem counterintuitive but eating less doesn't automatically equate to weight loss. In fact, it can create the opposite effect, resulting in weight gain because it triggers your body to conserve energy, not being able to predict when the next meal will come. In this case, the natural reaction is to decrease metabolic rate and burn less calories. Avoid this by eating at least five smaller, nutritious meals

each day and avoid skipping meals as much as possible. Experts at the Cleveland Clinic claim that eating smaller meals throughout the day will stabilize blood sugar levels and make our metabolism more efficient.[41] When deciding on which foods to eat, a good rule of thumb is to choose unsweetened versions of the foods you already enjoy, such as plain yogurt instead of a flavored one. Lastly, practice mindful eating. Avoid technology while you eat or eating directly out of packages, as you're likely going to consume a higher number of calories. Instead, eat with intention, enjoying your food. Contrary to what some of our moms used to say about having to finish what's on our plate, I say that you should give yourself permission to stop eating when you're no longer hungry.

2. Eat Protein and Healthy Fats with Every Meal: Protein and fat are the backbones of any healthy diet. Protein keeps you fuller longer, preventing pantry raids for snacks and supports muscle and brain health. If you're eating protein (plant or animal is fine) every time you eat, you'll live a healthier life. Healthy fats provide energy, support cell growth, protect organs, and are the pathway for your body to absorb vitamins A, D, E, and K. They also help with hormone production. So, ensure that each meal that you eat has a little bit of both protein and healthy fats. Great food choices to always have on hand that are high in fat and protein include avocados, nuts, olive oil, fish like salmon, and eggs. Good items to have in your pantry also include beans, chickpeas, lentils, artichokes, and tomatoes.
3. Hydrate: Drinking water will help keep

your blood sugar stable and also help curb your cravings. Very often, thirst is mistaken for hunger and we reach for a snack instead of water. Before you reach for a snack, always drink a glass of water first and give it at least five minutes. In addition to always having some water near you, also keep in mind that we can get some hydration from vegetables as well. Cucumber and lettuce are 96% water, tomato and celery both have 95% water content, and even broccoli is 90% water.[42] Those water-rich vegetables are also a great option to have nearby for when cravings hit.

Avoid the juices, blends, mix-ins, sodas, sweetened drinks (including specialty teas and coffees), and simply drink water as often as you can. Your goal should be to get an half an ounce of water for every pound you weigh—everyday (a full ounce if you're working out) but as a general rule of thumb, 60 ounces daily should be plenty.

4. Be Active: Fitness and nutrition are the one-two punch of a healthy lifestyle. You should strive to leave time each day for some kind of activity that gets your body moving. You'll never have to 'live in the gym' like an athlete (unless you want to), but you should be going for walks, playing sports, stretching, dancing, swimming, or even playing tag with your kids on a regular basis. We are living much more sedentary lives compared to our ancestors as many of us spend majority of our waking hours sitting down for both work and binge-watching relaxation time. A frequently quoted study in 2015 labelled prolonged

sitting as big of a threat to our health as smoking, leading to headlines like "your chair is killing you." Subsequent research in 13 studies noted that "those who sat for more than eight hours a day with no physical activity had a risk of dying similar to the risks of dying posed by obesity and smoking."[43]

At the very least, try to stand up every 30 minutes and move your body. By standing, an average of 50 extra calories is burned per hour in comparison to sitting. Standing 3 hours each day, five days per week adds up to 750 calories. Over the course of a year that adds up to 30,000 calories, which is almost 9 pounds.[44] Move your body naturally by standing and walking, but also carve out some sort of higher intensity workout at least for 30 minutes, 3 times per week. If you happen to feel that your energy tank is getting a little depleted, grab a bottle of water, a No Sugar Co. snack and go for a quick walk. It's the best way to boost up your energy and your mood. Your focus and dedication to your own well-being will push you farther than you ever dreamed!

5. Plan and Prepare: It is critical that you set yourself up for success. First, clean your environment from all added sugar foods, because if it's in the house, you are very likely going to eat it. There's nothing that can derail your no sugar goals like going to the grocery store without a plan. Make your list before you go to the store and keep your path on the perimeter where the fresh produce, healthy fats and protein are located. This will bypass the processed foods you no longer need. Also, when in a store, pay attention to labels. Check the sugar content and suggested serving sizes, which are often too small for a realistic meal. Avoid most packaged foods that have words ending in 'ose,' such as fructose, dextrose, and maltose, and look for syrups and juices on their ingredient list (see The many names of added sugars in Chapter 2). Eat before you shop or create your shopping lists as that will make you avoid choosing higher-calorie foods.[45] Ensure your snack drawer is stocked with No Sugar Co. alternatives, pack your fridge with plenty of pre chopped veggies and fruit and, when cooking, do it in batches so that the freezer is well stocked. If you plan ahead, you will make it a lot easier on yourself and more likely to reach your goals.

6. Go Green With Veggies: Strive to have leafy greens at least twice a day. Green veggies are among the best foods you can eat to improve your health and the No Sugar In Me lifestyle wholeheartedly supports eating your greens daily!

7. Set Realistic Goals: Be fair to yourself and your plans will see results. It's not wrong to want to see results quickly, but it won't do you any good if you let a lack of immediate change derail your progress. This is a lifestyle change. That means that you're going to get better each day. This isn't about a few weeks of eating a certain way to look better. This is about changing your life so you can look better, feel better, and live longer!

8. Sleep More: If you're the type to burn the candle at both ends, you're not helping your efforts to improve your health. Sleep is essential for your brain and body to repair and replenish, as well as maintain a healthy balance of blood sugar levels. There are a number of studies that show people who are sleep deprived consumed more calories, sugary foods, and sodas and fewer fruits and vegetables, compared to those who went to bed earlier and got between six to seven hours of rest.[46] In fact, just one night of getting only 4 hours of sleep can reduce insulin sensitivity and blood sugar levels.[47] The great news is that this pattern can be reversed with sufficient sleep in just one night.[48] Thus, aim for 6 to 7 hours of quality sleep each night.

The best tips for having higher quality sleep include: Ensure the room is pitch dark, avoid tech for the last hour of being awake, and turn the temperature down by a few degrees. If you must eat something a few hours before bedtime, try snacks that contain natural melatonin (a hormone that aids healthy sleep). This includes nuts like walnuts, peanuts and pistachios, goji berries, eggs, milk, or even oily fish like salmon and sardines.[49] Avoid heavy meals, spicy foods, caffeine, or alcohol that will likely interfere with your healthy sleep patterns.

9. Weigh Yourself Less: When I made the change, I stopped weighing myself. I didn't need a scale to tell me I felt better about myself and neither do you. Your weight will drop, your body will tighten up, and you'll look better each day, but your health will improve that much more.

10. Track Your Meals and Workouts:
Planning is key to all successful things but tracking your progress may be even more important. I always keep a log of what I eat and what I do for activity. It keeps me on task and mindful of my efforts in relation to my goals. As you get started, journal your initial eating habits without restrictions. Write down what you eat, when, and how often. After you have at least 2 days of information, review it. See how many meals you eat, when you snack, and when you feel that craving for sugar. That will help you identify and focus on what you would need to change. Also, note the time of day when your cravings hit. For most of us, our circadian rhythm, or internal clock, increases hunger and cravings for sweet and starchy foods in the evenings.[50] Eating larger meals, especially late at night, puts us at a higher risk of overeating and selecting unhealthy foods, according to researchers at Harvard University.[51] This is why we tend to crave the worst snacks at night. When you eat earlier and pack your diet with nutritious meals and snacks, you mitigate these cravings. Make sure you have the appropriate No Sugar Co. snacks and alternatives ready to go. Eat right every day and be active every day and you're on your way to a whole new you!

Quitting Immediately: What to Expect
You can decide to do gradual sugar reduction by applying the suggested quick steps above and that's entirely ok. If on the other hand, you decide that you want to break up with sugar immediately the way that I originally decided, I want you to be pre-pared for what to expect. There is a certain pattern that we will all experience as we eliminate added sugars out of our diets. The great news is that the toughest times are typically experienced only in the first 2 to 4 days. By the end of the first week, the majority of the people feel great and have a renewed sense of energy.

In my first few days, especially in days 2 and 3, I felt lethargic, unmotivated and even had headaches. This is entirely normal, and I want you to be prepared. How does that help? Well, let me give you an example. When I was serious about becoming a professional basketball player, I tried my best to always be prepared for anything on the court. However, if someone were to tell me all the plays of the opposing team before a game (I wish), I'd be ready for their game and know how to beat it with ease. Why am I telling you this? Because being prepared ensures an easier path to success. I'm being honest and telling you there are going to be difficult days and hours but knowing the challenge will be there should arm you with the resolve to weather any storm.

Another reason why I'm saying it at this stage is that at about three days or so after you've quit added sugar, the withdrawals will start kicking in. You might experience cravings, headaches, sore muscles, and emotionally feeling down. Exercise will help curb these feelings. Also, a magnesium supplement may come in handy. According to the National Institutes of Health, your daily recommended amount of Magnesium

(310 to 420mg per day) can help eliminate some of these symptoms and side effects.[52] If you don't want to take a supplement, you could also consider adding some spinach to your lunch and supper.

This is natural. This is just your body readjusting to new levels of dopamine. Remember, it had gotten used to those sugar highs. But you can work through it. At least now, you know it's coming, and you'll be prepared for the challenge just like I would have been if I had been given the opposing team's playbook.

Thankfully, those withdrawals will taper off within a week or so. Depending on how deep you were into the added sugar zone, it might take you slightly longer than a week. Just be kind to yourself during this time, stay hydrated, and work through our craving crusher tips listed earlier in this chapter.

One and a half weeks after you quit, you'll start to feel great. If you take the time to observe how you feel in comparison to your previous state of being, you'll notice that you'll be more active, have a cleaner, healthier energy about your daily routine and feel more tranquil in your world. Give yourself a big pat on the back at this point. You've battled through an intense biological, physiological event and come through it on top.

One month after you quit, you'll find that your life is totally different. Your desire for sugary desserts will have vanished. And you may even find that your cravings have changed entirely. When this first happened to me, I almost couldn't believe it. I was talking to a friend on the phone about my no sugar change, and he asked about whether or not I actually missed my old lifestyle and approach to food. I shocked myself when I answered, honestly, that I didn't crave that sugary stuff anymore.

A year after you've quit, your health will have improved incredibly. Your energy levels will rise and stay consistent, your skin will be clearer, hair fuller, and general disposition and mood will improve dramatically. Your body will now be adjusted to functioning more on whole foods. Because it no longer has to store all that added sugar as fat, you'll also drop weight. But beyond weight loss, you'll be more healthy and energized, and you'll have better, deeper and restful sleep. Funny how these things all go hand-in-hand, isn't it?

I intentionally didn't devise this book or movement as a diet because they are often too restrictive or too complex to follow. This isn't about counting calories or points or trips to the gym. Diets and plans like that generally don't work long term anyway. Also, this isn't about starving yourself. This is about the easy steps that will lead to healthy food choices and lifestyle. Find your own new normal for what you eat daily and say it loudly: No Sugar: I Am Sweet Enough!

Chapter 05

KETO MADE SIMPLE: NO SUGAR AND KETO DIET

There are so many popular diets out there, some of which you may have tried out yourself – Intermittent Fasting, Atkins, Weight Watchers, South Beach diet and the list goes on and on. Do you know the ONE thing that all diets have in common? **All diets recommend not eating refined sugar!** So, to reinforce my earlier point, if you just cut down the amount of sugar you eat, you're likely going to see a difference in your waistline.

Having said that, if you wanted to take it a step further, one of the most popular diets in North America that addresses not only weight loss but also claims to help with several other health concerns is Keto Diet. I've had so many friends and family members try keto and saw first-hand when done right, what an effective diet this is. Some of my friends lost more than 50lbs while on

it! We will focus on this diet specifically as it is intrinsically linked to the elimination of sugar and its overall benefits on health. Thus, in this chapter, we will look at keto diet and provide tips on how to be successful with it.

History of Keto

The Keto diet isn't just the latest fad and has quite a cool story worth knowing. It's been around for more than 100 years, when created by modern day physicians to help treat epilepsy in children in 1920s[53]. The renewed interest and popularity of this diet started in 1994 by a Hollywood producer Jim Abrahams. He became a big proponent of the keto diet, as his son's severe epilepsy was improved once he was put on keto. Jim created a foundation to provide funding for keto research and produced a movie about it "Do No Harm", starring

Meryl Streep. Since then, keto diet has been gaining popularity as celebrities began endorsing it and over the last decade, it became one of the most searched diets on google[54]. Read on to find out why!

What is Keto?

In simplest terms, keto diet recommends consuming high healthy fats, low net carbs and moderate protein. This change in your diet will turn your body from using carbs as its source of fuel to using fat, eventually getting your body into a state of ketosis. When in ketosis, your body will burn fat instead of carbs, and thus inducing weight loss.

Unlike with most other diets, keto diet is very satiating as people generally feel quite full when eating high levels of healthy fats. However, what does make it challenging is that keto is much more restrictive in carbs compared to other diets. In fact, it is recommended that daily carb intake should be capped at only 50g per day, which is less than a cup of rice or pasta, and really easily consumed through just a few pieces of fruit.

Why are sugar and carbs so restricted on keto diet? Well, **every gram of sugar is considered a carb**, which is why both of those categories are not recommended while on keto. In other words, avoid carbs, avoid sugar.

Instead of carbs and sugar, you would focus on foods high in fat and moderate in protein (for a complete list and shopping suggestions, scroll down).

KETO RATIO MICRONUTRIENT INTAKE	vs	USDA RECOMMENDED MICRONUTRIENT INTAKE
70% Fat		20% Fat
20% Protein		30% Protein
10% Carbohydrates[55]		50% Carbohydrates

This diet does require discipline but when done right, it also provides visible results in a relatively short amount of time. One of the hardest things I experienced while on keto was finding foods with low net carbs that are also healthy and indulgent to eat as treats. That is why many No Sugar Co products are keto friendly and work well with your keto goals.

Benefits of Ketosis

As mentioned, one of the reasons why keto is gaining such popularity is that it's an effective weight-loss solution and yet, you won't be as hungry as you normally would be on many other diets. A reduced appetite on keto is mainly due to an increase in fat consumption. Have you ever been hungry after eating a ten-ounce New York steak? I haven't.

While most people are using keto diet as an efficient solution for weight loss, its effects on several health conditions including diabetes, Alzheimer's, headaches and even sleep disorders are being evaluated. While scientific research is still underway, anecdotally, many people are claiming the benefits they personally experienced while on keto including weight loss, increased energy, moderated inflammation, blood sugar, insulin, and cholesterol levels.[56] This all sounds quite incredible, so you may ask, "how does a ketogenic diet do all this"?

Well for one, it helps you lose abdominal or visceral fat which tends to get lodged around the internal organs. Why is that so important? Excess visceral fat squeezes your internal organs making it harder for them to function, which can result in a myriad of serious health conditions such as type 2 diabetes and heart disease.[57]

Also, given that keto diet is low in carbohydrates, it can also elevate the good cholesterol (HDL) and lower the bad (LDL) cholesterol. Many people who are diagnosed as pre-diabetic or diabetic have seen significant reduction of their blood sugar levels after going on keto. If this applies to you and you are considering keto diet, certainly consult your physician.

To sum it all up, keto diet can certainly help in the following areas:
- Decrease risk of high blood pressure
- Decrease levels of abdominal fat
- Improve blood sugar / insulin levels
- Improve cholesterol levels
- Improve inflammation

Keto Flu and How To Fight It

While keto may sound like an amazing diet, if you are considering it, you should also be aware of the potential side effects. While the long-term effects are still being studied and come with their own warning label,

one of the most frequently experienced issues is commonly known as keto flu. It describes the symptoms some people feel especially in the first week of their keto diet, while they are retraining their metabolism and moving their body into ketosis. Symptoms of the keto flu include headaches, slumps in energy, agitation, constipation, difficulties concentrating, muscle aches and extreme sugar cravings. These symptoms typically occur in days 3 to 5 of your diet and unlike with a regular flu, they are not contagious. Good news is that they taper off by the end of your first week.

While you can brave through it knowing that it won't last forever, you can also offset some of the pain by being well prepared and addressing the challenges head on.

Tip 1: Increase your salt and water consumption
As you enter ketosis, one of the ways your body will respond is by pushing out sodium (i.e., salt) through urine. Thus, you may find yourself going to the bathroom more often than usual. To offset that, it is important that you consume more water than you normally would and compliment it with added salt. Try drinking a glass of water with half a teaspoon of salt whenever you experience one of the keto-flu symptoms. You can also drink salted bone broth, chicken or beef stock with bullion and perhaps add a bit of salted butter for elevated fat levels. The symptoms will likely fade away 15 to 30 minutes thereafter.

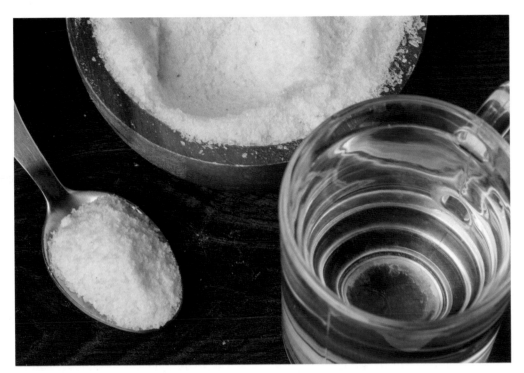

Tip 2: Eat LOTS of healthy fats.

It is important that as you transition into keto diet, you do not restrict your fat and caloric intake. If you combine decrease in carbs with a decrease in calories, your body may be triggered to go into starvation mode. Instead, ensure that you eat foods that are high in fat especially in the beginning and do not count calories.

Do note that there is a difference between inclusion of healthy fats versus saturated or trans fats. The best sources of healthy fats include avocados, olive and avocado oils, nuts and nut butters, seeds, and fatty fish. On the other hand, be sure to limit the amount of saturated fat in the diet and avoid even small intakes of trans fats which can be found in deep fried or fast food, shortening and margarine. Ensure that you are well prepared for this transition and have a fridge and pantry stocked with foods that you can eat like nuts, butters, eggs and of course, some of our keto treats for those sneaky sugar cravings.

Let your appetite guide you and eat keto-friendly foods until you feel satisfied. Try to eat slowly and mindfully to avoid over-eating and know that once your body is in ketosis, your appetite will also slow down.

Tip 3: Don't exert yourself

You are training your body to use a different fuel as a source of energy, that is, use fat instead of carbs. Expect that the transition may be strenuous for your body, and you will likely experience slumps in your energy levels initially. Thus, try not to have any highly intensive workouts planned for the first few weeks. Instead, try to incorporate gentle movement such as stretching, walking or yoga. Research does show that energy levels do recover between weeks 4 and 6 so keep that in mind as you plan your exercise routine.

What Do You Eat on the Keto Diet?

To prepare yourself for the keto diet, start by making small adjustments at every meal. For example, enjoy a hamburger patty wrapped in a Bibb or Romaine lettuce leaf. Order a salad or eat vegetables in place of French fries. In place of a baked potato, enjoy cauliflower rice tossed in olive oil, pepper, and garlic, sprinkled with Parmesan cheese. Start pushing the carbs and sugar out of your life gradually and focus on moderate protein and healthy fats.[58] This works best when your adjust slowly. Making drastic dietary changes immediately can make the transition that much harder.

When you're ready to start, the meals couldn't be simpler. From the list below, create your own meals that let you hit the 70% fat, 20% protein and 10% carbs ratio in each meal and you'll see results.

Net Carbs

You've probably also heard the term 'net carbs' before, especially if you've been trying to make changes to your diet. This is a term that's used to tell you exactly how many total carbohydrates your food has, minus the fiber and sugar substitutes. Why is this important? That number of carbs is the actual amount of carbs your body is taking in and converting to glucose to use as energy and potentially stored as belly fat if you've eaten too much. Your body can't absorb fiber so it can't be put through that conversion process. Here's a simple way to calculate the net carbs of anything you'll eat with an example:

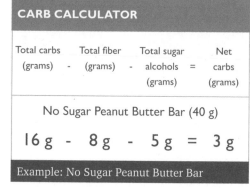

CARB CALCULATOR			
Total carbs (grams) -	Total fiber (grams) -	Total sugar alcohols (grams) =	Net carbs (grams)
No Sugar Peanut Butter Bar (40 g)			
16 g -	8 g -	5 g =	3 g
Example: No Sugar Peanut Butter Bar			

There are a number of free keto calculators that will help you estimate your net carb consumption so do look those up if you decided to give this diet a try.

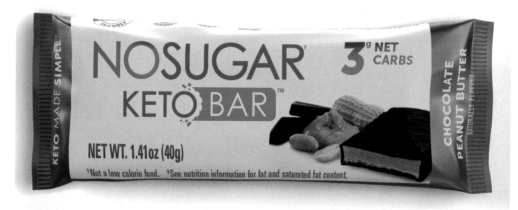

Lastly, note that carbohydrates are sugars that come in two forms: Simple and complex. Complex carbohydrates are present in foods like fruits and veggies, beans, leafy greens, whole wheat bread, and potatoes. Simple carbohydrates are found in low nutritional foods like syrups, sugary drinks, chocolate bars, bagels, white bread, store bought pasta, and table sugar—the worst offenders of which being comprised of added, refined sugar like the packaged foods across your grocery store. Simple carbohydrates can produce a spike in blood glucose, often producing a 'sugar rush' while providing the body with a short-lasting source of energy. Complex carbs don't do that because they are balanced by the fiber, vitamins, and nutrients that they come with naturally.[59]

Quick Keto Swaps

The thought of eating a meal without potatoes, rice, pasta or tortillas may sound intimidating at first, but there are some ways to follow a keto diet without carbs, and by extension, sugar. Here are seven quick and easy swaps to follow a ketogenic diet without sugar, while not sacrificing what you want to eat:

- Make rice out of vegetables like cauliflower, broccoli or Brussels sprouts. Simply grate the veggies, toss with olive oil and season with garlic and herbs and you won't miss the rice at all.

- Wrap your burgers or sandwiches in Boston Bibb or Romaine lettuce leaves instead of a bun or tortilla.

- In place of potatoes, choose lower-carbohydrate vegetables such as sweet potatoes, squash, or turnips.

- Spiralize vegetables like zucchini and squash in place of noodles for pasta.

- In place of artificial creamers, look for unsweetened plant-based milk such as almond, oat, soy or coconut milk.

- When it comes to dessert, opt for dark chocolate, but be sure to look for at least 70% cocoa and minimal added sugar.

- If you're in search of a healthy and indulgent snack, of course I would recommend our No Sugar Company's Keto products (sorry I cannot help it)!

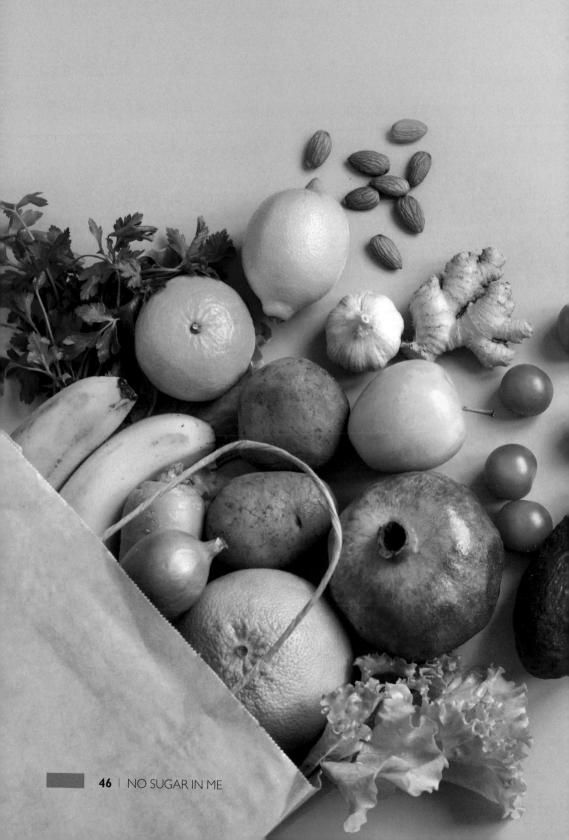

Keto Grocery Shopping List

PROTEINS

	Eggs
	Fish and Seafood (salmon, albacore tuna, mackerel, shrimp and sardines)
	Poultry and Beef

NO cold cuts or processed meats

FATS AND OILS

	Butter and heavy cream
	Extra-virgin olive oil
	Coconut oil

NO margarine

FRUITS AND VEGETABLES

	Low-Carbohydrate Vegetables (bell peppers, cauliflower, broccoli, green beans, spinach, zucchini, asparagus and celery)
	Berries (strawberries, blueberries, and raspberries)
	Avocado

NO potatoes, corn, bananas or most other fresh or dried fruit. No beans of any kind, peas, or lentils

NUTS AND SEEDS

	Nuts and Seeds (almonds, brazil nuts, cashews, walnuts, macadamia nuts, pecans, pistachios, ground flaxseed, chia seed, sesame, or pumpkin seeds)
	Ground flaxseed or chia seeds
	Unsweetened nut butters – peanut butter is allowed

NO flavored or glazed nuts, no peanuts

DAIRY

	Feta cheese
	Cheddar cheese
	Cottage Cheese

NO milk, non-fat yogurt or dairy-based ice cream (keto varieties can be found)

CONDIMENTS AND SNACKS

	Avocado
	Full-fat mayonnaise
	Vinegar
	Keto-safe snacks – variety of the options in this category is growing daily

NO milk, non-fat yogurt or dairy-based ice cream (keto varieties can be found)

NO traditional snack foods such as potato chips, pretzels and crackers

BAKED GOODS

	Keto bread only

NO other baked goods, pastas or any other grains (no rice, no oatmeal)

BEVERAGES

	Water (still or unflavored sparkling)
	Unsweetened Almond, Coconut or Oat Milk
	Tea
	Coffee

NO soft drinks, lemonade, juice or anything with sugars

Keto and Exercise

In order to get optimal results while on keto or any other diet, I highly recommend complimenting it with exercise. When implementing a change in your dietary habits and combining it with exercise or body movement regime, you will prevent plateaus when it comes to weight loss and instead, expedite it.

You need to move your body every single day. Full stop. Stand up every hour. Walk 10,000 steps. Or if you can't aim that high, walk 5,000. Do what you can but push yourself and increase your goals gradually. As humans, we are built to move, and while you burn fat while on ketogenic diet, combining it with exercise can help improve the speed of your weight loss.

Some evidence suggests that when it comes to keto, not all exercise is the same. For one, keto diet may not be ideal for high-intensity workouts that require short bursts of energy, such as weightlifting or high-intensity aerobics which are usually fueled by energy from carbs. Instead, keto diet seems better suited for steady-state exercise like powerwalking, jogging and cycling at a consistent pace. Because ketosis relies on burning fat instead of carbs, a body in ketosis is also likely to feel less energy bursts but burn calories faster than someone on a different diet would during the exact same exercise.[60]

Along the same lines, it is also claimed that keto diet is better for maintaining muscle mass rather than building it. Thus, when you've committed to this diet, you can expect improved endurance for steady-pace exercises, muscle recovery, and increased fat burning from your workouts.[61]

Hitting Pause if Needed

Plateaus in your weight loss efforts can be frustrating and there are many factors that can contribute to a stall in reaching your goal. The reason people lose so much weight on a keto diet is because it is hard to overeat when so much of your diet is comprised of fat and protein. Although it works, it isn't easy to maintain.

There are times when you may need to take a break from the reduction in calories and carbohydrates. The human brain is designed to monitor your weight and elicit processes to keep you from losing weight too fast so you can survive times of famine. While that is hard to do, your mind and body don't know you are going on a diet, and those defensive processes can kick in at full force, derailing your efforts.[62]

If you want to stay on track, a great method is to plan a cheat day. While it is counter intuitive, a study done in the International Journal of Obesity discovered that taking a 'diet break' can be very effective in losing weight rather than maintaining a constant reduction in calories.[63] By taking a 'diet break,' you can help keep your body from decreasing its resting energy expenditure and experience more consistent weight loss, busting through any plateau.

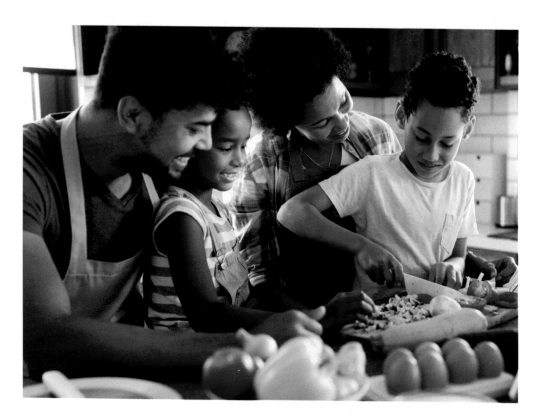

One simple truth that a lot of people don't tell you about the keto diet is that it can be extremely difficult to stay on it and is an unlikely long-term lifestyle choice for many of the people. I've found that the keto dietary approach is best when it's used in cycles. This gives you the benefit of expediting your fat burning potential but once it tapers off, you can and ease back into a No Sugar In Me lifestyle without the inevitable pitfalls that come from ending a diet and going back to poor dietary choices.

Key Takeaways

Although very popular and effective, keto diet can be challenging as let's be honest, carbs and sugars are not the easiest things to give up. Having said that, a number of responsible companies have been working really hard to find appropriate substitutes that would make that experience easier. You can find all kinds of tools in place like keto sticks to identify if your body is in ketosis, calculators, and keto-friendly recipes. Also note that gone are the days where keto products need to taste dry and chalky. Instead, you can expect an ever-growing category of tasty and indulgent food items that will make you feel excited about this journey to continue to evolve over the coming years. For more on what's coming from our own No Sugar Company kitchen, skip ahead to Chapter 8!

Chapter 06

HOW TO START AND STRIVE

Whenever you start a new approach to how you eat, workout, and even live your life, it's important to have an entry point so you can find your footing as quickly as possible. I know that the toughest part of this new lifestyle is going to be adapting to what you can and should not be eating. With that in mind, I devised the following quick-start plan so you can make the first week as easy as possible!

You'll start each day with a high-protein breakfast followed by a sensible snack a couple hours later. Then, you'll have lunch, following that up with a snack a couple hours later. Your final meal of the day is a sensible dinner that is high in protein and healthy fats. After that, a few hours before bedtime, you can choose to have another sensible snack if you are hungry.

What you will notice from the meals and snacks below is that I chose not to list calories, fat, sugars, or carbohydrates. This is not a diet. It is a lifestyle. It is a reset of your approach to food. As such, you should be focusing on the real, natural ingredients that have no sugar added. Enjoy the food and coast through this week and your body will crave these kinds of meals going forward—all without calculating any caloric data.

Another great part about this approach is that you will choose which breakfast, lunch, dinner and snacks you eat every day from this list of options.

More recipes will also be available in our app as well as future updates of the book. Create your meal plan in Appendix E!

Breakfast

There's actually a large body of research that supports the claim that breakfast is the most important meal of the day. Breakfast replenishes the energy and nutrients in your body. Eating breakfast will boost your energy levels and restore glycogen levels, which will rev up your metabolism. You might have been skipping breakfast in the past but that has to stop.

Breakfast Option 1: Fruit Parfait

1 cup Greek yogurt with 1 cup mixed berries

Breakfast Option 2: Oatmeal

1 cup cooked oatmeal with 1 cup unsweetened milk and 1 ounce of raisins or a half apple (mixed in or on the side)

Breakfast Option 3: Eggs

2 eggs (any style you prefer) and an orange.

Breakfast Option 4: 'No Sugar Co. KetO's (coming soon)

Snacks

While you decide when you have your snacks each day, this quick-start expects you'll have a minimum of two each day, but no more than three. The optimum approach is to have a snack between breakfast and lunch and then another between lunch and supper. If you're hungry in the mid-evening, you can opt to have another snack at that time. The goal is to keep you going throughout the day with what you need, never overeating and always making sure you have the fuel to accomplish everything you set out to do for the day.

Snack Option 1: Fresh Fruit

Again, the choice is yours, but you can't go wrong with mixed berries.

1 cup mixed berries (blueberries, strawberries and cranberries are ideal). This is an excellent choice for your mid evening snack after dinner because cranberries have been proven to be a sleep aid.

Snack Option 2: Veggie Dip

1 cup celery and /or carrots with ¼ cup hummus

Snack Option 3: Sweet and Savory

1 skim milk mozzarella cheese stick with a handful of grapes

Snack Option 4: No Sugar Co. snacks: Cups/bombs, bars, clusters, or krax

Lunch

The middle of the day usually brings about the most hunger. We are programmed to need food from years of feasting at that time and this plan delivers healthy meals to satisfy that hunger. Because lunch tends to be a meal we eat away from home, the goal of the following meals is to be as simple, mobile, and nutritious as possible.

If you stick with these meals and avoid the temptation of grabbing something somewhat 'healthy' from a restaurant or fast-food eatery, you'll feel great and have energy straight through to the end of the day!

Lunch Option 1: Chicken

6 to 8 ounces broiled diced chicken with 1 ounce cheddar cheese and half cup of celery. You could also do this by substituting baked ham instead of chicken.

Lunch Option 2: Eggs

2 hard-boiled eggs with a cup of cherry tomatoes

Lunch Option 3: Tuna

6 ounces of tuna (water drained from the can), with half an avocado and 1 piece of whole wheat toast.

Lunch Option 4: Lettuce Wrap

Two leaves of lettuce or cabbage with shredded chicken or tuna with an avocado slice in each. You should aim for about 6 ounces of protein over the two lettuce wraps.

Dinner

With work asking more from most of us than ever before, and commute times at their worst, it is hard to buck the growing trend of eating later in the evening. With that in mind, it's even more critical that you eat a healthy meal for dinner, so you aren't packing in added sugars, saturated fats, and artificial flavors into your body. The following meals are easy to make, can be pre-made when you have more time, and deliver a lot of flavor and nutrients.

Dinner Option 1: Salmon

1 6 ounce filet of salmon, grilled or broiled with half cup of asparagus and a half sliced tomato.

Dinner Option 2: Steak

5 ounce sirloin steak, grilled or broiled with half sweet potato, baked, and cup of mixed greens, topped with one tablespoon of balsamic vinaigrette.

Dinner Option 3: Chicken Fajitas

7 ounces of boneless, skinless chicken breast, sliced into strips, sauteed on a skillet with diced onions, peppers and tomatoes.

Dinner Option 4: Your Choice Salad

Create your own salad with your choice of protein from the above meals (up to 7 ounces, but no less than 4) with two cups of mixed greens, a quarter avocado, 4 cherry tomatoes, 3 tablespoons of balsamic vinaigrette and a hard-boiled egg (optional).

Can You Use Spices?

This question often comes up when anyone is about to start a new meal plan. Yes, you can use spices, but you should never let spices be the focus of the taste on your plate. Everything you will eat in this plan has great, natural flavor. Loading it up with salt, pepper or sauces will only bury that flavor and taint your appreciation of the meal you prepared. Here are some suggestions for spices so you can enhance your meals without losing flavor along with a few that have been shown to have a very positive effect on our blood sugar levels.

Salt: While you certainly can add a small dash of salt to any of the meals listed on this plan, you shouldn't rely on salt for flavor. A little goes a long way. If you feel you need more than a shake or two of a salt shaker, try freshly cracked pepper instead and some lemon juice.

Lemon Juice: Consider lemon juice your best friend when it comes to this plan. Use it on your meals and in your drinks. It adds natural flavor and helps curb your appetite.

Chili Flakes: You should stay away from using hot sauce on your meals. They are often packed with sodium and preservatives. Instead, use chili flakes to up the heat on your plate.

Oregano: A light dusting of oregano can really pop in some flavor to a salad, or with any of the proteins you are eating on this plan. Add about a teaspoon or less and you've got a nice complement to your meal.

Other spices to consider: Turmeric, cinnamon, mint, ginger, mustard, fenugreek seed, and cumin as they've all been deemed as being diabetes-friendly due to their effect on blood sugar levels.

Staying Hydrated

I strongly believe that water is your best choice. This is a no sugar lifestyle, so you obviously can't be drinking sodas, sugar-packed coffee drinks, and the like, but you can have black coffee or tea with some stevia, water with lemon, and freshly squeezed fruit juices (to avoid derailing your progress with drinks that are pre-bottled and packed with sugar).
Hydration is key in any dietary change. This is why your water consumption is the most important factor when it comes to what you drink and when going through this quick-start.

Sipping on water throughout the day will keep you hydrated, your mind clear, and your muscles ready for any challenge. Couple that with coffee and tea and you should have all you need.

Before you Begin

Compared with the 'diets' out there, this one-week plan is actually quite easy. You're getting plenty of food and all the nutrients your body should require. However, no healthy lifestyle shift should be considered without the addition of a once daily multivitamin (not that sugar-filled gummy version though). This will ensure that you are not lacking on any vitamins and minerals.

Simple Swaps

What you'll learn from this lifestyle is that you truly are in charge of your choices. I'm not telling you what you have to eat, what you have to avoid, when you have to work out, or what products to buy.

Instead, the No Sugar In Me lifestyle is a framework you should aim to live within. That's why this book offers guidance and suggestions, rather than strict rules. However, I know better than most that sometimes you just need a quick and easy guide to follow when it comes to some of the most common dietary mistakes people make. Below you'll find a list of foods you may think you want and the swaps that can satisfy and stay on track.

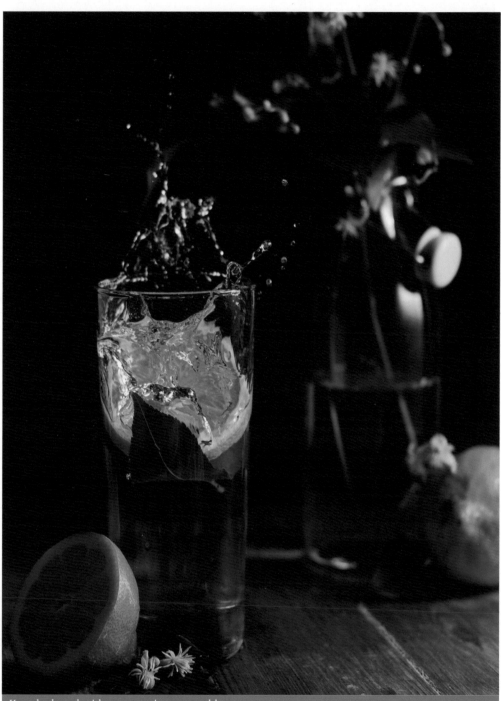

Keep hydrated with great tasting, natural lemon water.

1. Want: Bread

Bread is the backbone of so many meals. Beyond the sandwiches, burgers, and pizzas, some people simply crave bread on its own. As a staple of diets since its inception, it's hard to address the truth about bread, but it's packed with sugar, carbs, and fat. You can do better.

Nutrition facts of 2 slices of White Bread
Sugar 4 grams
Calories 140
Fat 2.5 grams
Carbohydrates 29 grams

SWAP: Boston Bibb Lettuce

If you haven't swapped bread for lettuce wraps yet, you're missing out. Adding in a crunch to any sandwich is always smart, but with this swap you're also dropping calories, fat, carbs, and sugar. This is a no brainer.

Nutrition facts for a serving of Boston Bibb Lettuce
Sugar 1 grams
Calories 11
Fat 0 grams
Carbohydrates 2 grams

2. Want: Cola

While I haven't touched a sugar-filled cola in years, I admit to drinking it at least a couple times a week growing up. I know it's hard to avoid soft drinks with the way most eateries are approaching food these days, but this is one drink you have to swap out if you want to live a No Sugar In Me lifestyle.

Nutrition Facts of Cola (20 ounce serving)
Sugar 65 grams
Calories 240
Carbohydrates 65 grams

Swap: Soda Water with a Lemon Slice or No Sugar Co JOYBURST (coming soon)

Let's face it, a lot of the urge to drink a soda is the crispness of the soda water and added flavor. A much better solution than the typical sugar-packed soda are the JOYBURST natural energy water from No Sugar Co. If you're in a pinch and you've run out, soda water with your choice of fruit (lemon, lime, orange, berries, kiwi etc.) along with some stevia can hit the same spot as well.

Nutrition Facts of No Sugar Co JOYBURST
Sugar 0 grams
Calories 0 grams
Net Carbohydrates 0 grams

3. Want: Low-Fat Yogurt

Yogurt used to be such a healthy snack. Now, it's become a sugary treat with dubious health-related promises. Look at nearly half of the yogurt at your local grocery store and you're bound to see the label "Low Fat." This may sound good, but it opens the door for empty calories, added sugar and a host of colors and additives.

Nutrition Facts on 6 ounces of Low-Fat Yogurt
Sugar 12 grams
Calories 90
Fat 0 grams
Protein 9 grams

Swap: Plain Greek Yogurt

Packed with protein, low in fat and sugar, all while tasting like the creamy snack yogurt was always intended to be? Sounds like a smart swap to me. In fact, you could even consider this as a swap for frozen dessert (No Sugar Keto Frozen Dessert Coming Soon). Bonus: You can add in nuts, diced up fruit, or some stevia to match your taste.

Nutrition Facts on 5 ounces of Plain Greek Yogurt
Sugar 2 grams
Calories 80
Fat 2 gram
Protein 12 grams

4. Want: Regular Coffee with cream and sugar

Somewhere along the way, society dubbed a regular coffee to be a serving of coffee accompanied with one cream and two packets of sugar. That made a healthy drink into one you need to miss.

Nutrition Facts of a Regular Coffee with cream and sugar.
Sugar 26 grams
Calories 190
Fat 9 grams
Carbohydrate 29 grams

Swap: Home Brewed Coffee

Nutrition Facts of Home Brew Coffee
Sugar 0 grams
Calories 2
Fat 0 grams
Carbohydrates 0 grams

5. Want: Candy Peanut Butter Cups

Unlike the typical candy bar, this one comes in cups and some people even think it's healthier than others because of the peanut butter. No matter what benefits could come from actual peanut butter, the added sugar in this snack far outweighs any benefit (real or perceived).

Nutrition Facts of Candy Peanut Butter Cup (21 gram serving)
Sugar 11 grams
Calories 110
Fat 7 grams
Carbohydrates 12 grams
Protein 3 grams

Swap: No Sugar Co. Keto Cups/Bombs

If you're looking for a more direct swap, you won't find one. These cups have the chocolate and peanut butter flavors you're looking for without the sugar. The taste is revved way up by the quality ingredients, specifically the dark chocolate and the healthy fats!

Nutrition Facts on the Peanut Butter No Sugar Keto Cup (17 gram serving)
Sugar 0 grams
Calories 70
Fat 8 grams
Net Carbohydrates 1 gram
Protein 1 gram

6. Want: Spaghetti Sauce

Store-bought sauces are a bad idea for anyone looking to limit sugars from their diet. That goes for spaghetti sauce, salad

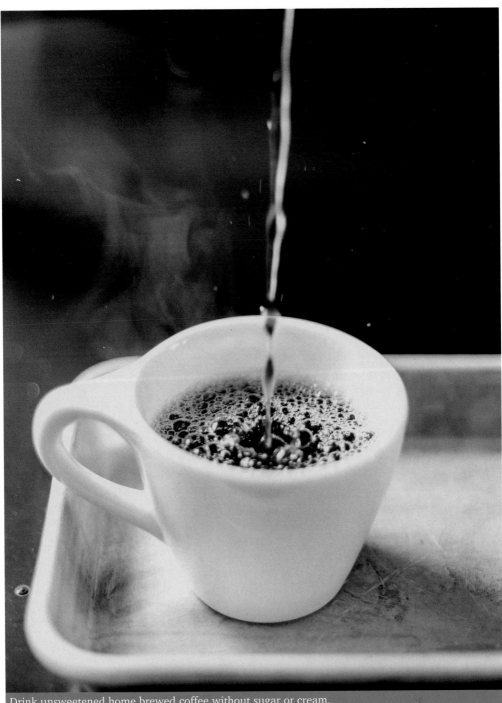

Drink unsweetened home brewed coffee without sugar or cream.

dressings, and even gravy. The reason I'm calling out spaghetti sauces is that they usually pack in a lot of sugar in an effort to provide flavor, which only exposes their lack of fresh ingredients.

Nutrition Facts on 1 cup of Traditional Store Brand Sauce
Sugar 16 grams
Calories 120
Fat 2 grams
Carbohydrates 22 grams

Swap: Homemade Sauce
You can't beat homemade tomato sauce. All you have to do is purée a couple of small tomatoes, add oregano, garlic, salt, and pepper to taste and let it sauté for about 20 minutes. It's simple, it tastes better, and it isn't packed with sugar and preservatives.

Nutrition Facts on Homemade Tomato Sauce
Natural Sugar 5 grams
Calories 32
Fat 1 gram
Carbohydrates 7 grams

7. Want: Chocolate Milk
This was one of my favorites growing up. I even remember being told that chocolate milk was a healthy option for athletes. Sure, there are some redeeming factors in chocolate milk like vitamin D and protein, but the sugar content can't be overlooked—especially when non-flavored milk has so much less.

Nutrition Facts on 1 cup of Chocolate Milk

Sugar 49 grams
Calories 570
Fat 23 grams
Carbohydrates 50 grams
Protein 9.3 grams

Swap: Unsweetened Almond Milk with Stevia and Cocoa Powder
I totally get the desire for a tall, cool glass of chocolate milk, but there's another way to get that fix. Mix stevia and some dark chocolate cocoa powder with some unsweetened almond milk and you won't sacrifice your diet.

Nutrition Facts on 1 cup Unsweetened Almond Milk with Stevia and Cocoa Powder
Sugar 0 grams
Calories 30
Fat 2.5 grams
Net Carbs 0 grams
Protein 1 grams

8. Want: Your Favorite Cereal
The childhood taste of your favorite breakfast cereal can't be denied, and neither can its high sugar and carb content. While it may seem like a good idea in the morning, most cereals list sugar as the highest content ingredient and they should not be a morning ritual for anyone living the No Sugar In Me lifestyle.

Nutrition Facts on 1 cup of your favorite cereal.
Sugar 12 grams
Calories 100
Fat 1.5 grams
Protein 3 grams

Swap: Large Flake Oatmeal or No Sugar Co. KetO's Cereal (Coming Soon)

The breakfast cereal you grew up with isn't all it's cracked up to be. Grow up and eat some oats for breakfast. As well as being a no sugar option, it also packs in 15 grams of protein per cup. Also, be on the lookout for No Sugar Co KetO's cereal that will satisfy any morning craving, nostalgic or otherwise.

Nutrition Facts on 1 cup of Large Flake Oatmeal
Sugar 0 grams

Calories 360
Fat 2 grams
Protein 15 grams

Nutrition Facts on 3/4 cup of No Sugar Co. KETO's
Sugar 0
Calories 110-120
Fat 4-5g
Net Carbohydrates 4-5grams
Protein 8-10 grams

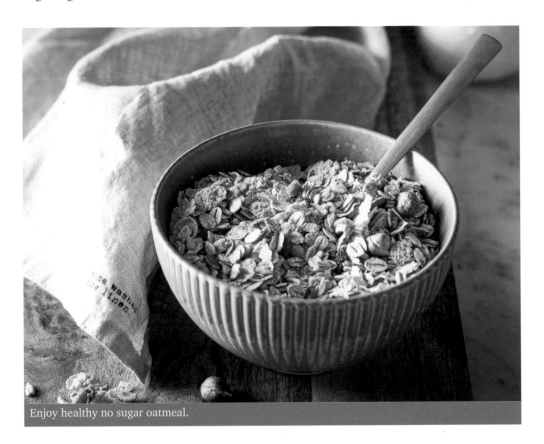

Enjoy healthy no sugar oatmeal.

Chapter 07

NO SUGAR KIGS KIDS

This chapter is very personal to me as I am the proud father of Summer and Ivy, who are 7 and 5 years old. They are the reason why I wanted to create more awareness about refined sugar and create healthier options for kids without processed sugar. This is written not only for parents and caregivers, but also for grandparents, cool aunts and uncles, older siblings, and anyone who interacts with or looks after our future generation.

On the following pages, I will highlight some concerning health research directly related to our kids, elevating the importance of setting the right eating habits as early as possible. I will also offer some advice on what worked in our home along with my thoughts on how to speak about sugar, parties, and even school lunches.

Much like with our quick-start recommendations in Chapter 5, depending on where you are in your own nutritional journey, it is likely that you are already following some of these recommendations, which is great. If not, feel free to experiment by choosing a few of the tips and test them out yourself. The honest truth is that as caregivers, we are always learning and it may feel like things are perfect one day, only to have things go sideways the very next. Consider this as a safe place for discovery as you'll hopefully learn a few good things and find what works best for you and your family.

I strongly believe that if a child has a positive relationship with food, it will set them up on the right path not only health-wise, but it will also act as a building block for

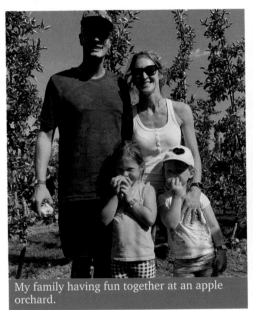
My family having fun together at an apple orchard.

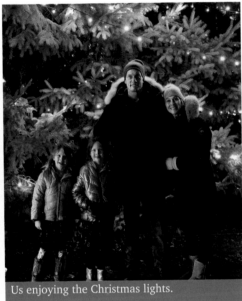
Us enjoying the Christmas lights.

their confidence and positive body image. This is a very tall order that requires our collective effort.

Why It Matters: Early Years

As early as six to seven years ago, when we had our first daughter, my wife and I noticed that even baby food contained added sugar. At the time, we made every effort to make our own baby food at home without realizing how much of an uphill battle it would continue to be for the coming years. Ironically, the first time our oldest daughter, Summer, had refined sugar was when she broke her arm and visited a doctor who gave her a popsicle for "being a brave girl."

Yes, inevitably all children will be introduced to refined sugar and that's ok but delaying that introduction for as long as possible is something that science supports. Allowing children's tastebuds to develop preference for natural foods for as long as possible really does matter.

A recent study published in the *Journal of Experimental Biology,* showed that food consumed by kids under the age of six, directly correlates to their health for the rest of their lives. Researchers were themselves surprised at the extent of influence the early years have on our microbiomes and subsequent exercise habits, that they concluded that even if people change dietary habits after childhood, they may not be able to shake the negative effects of a bad childhood diet. What does that really mean? The researchers argue that it's not an issue of 'You are what you eat' anymore but rather 'You are what you ate as a child.'[64]

Regulators are beginning to take notice and, however slowly, implement changes. Just last year, in July of 2020, the USDA released a report making a clear recommendation for the very first time to: "Avoid all foods and beverages with added sugars during the first 2 years of life…[as] the energy in such products is likely to displace energy from nutrient-dense foods, increasing the risk of nutrient inadequacies." The American Heart Association is also now actively supporting and promoting that added sugar should be avoided before age 2. It's a small but critically important first step to ensure our children are given a strong start in their early years.[65]

Adolescents

If you are past the toddler years, challenges to eat healthy get tougher in some ways. According to the American Heart Association, children between 2 and 18 years old should have less than 25 grams or 6 teaspoons of processed sugar daily.[66] They're precise about the number, and also the distinction of 'processed sugar' so parents don't tell their kids to avoid eating healthy foods like fruits and vegetables (which is where we should all be getting natural sugar from).

How quickly can you get up to (or past) 25 grams? Consider this:
• Low-fat yogurt cup can have up to 45 grams
• Leading kids nutrition bar has 10 grams
• Leading brand cereals have 10-12 grams

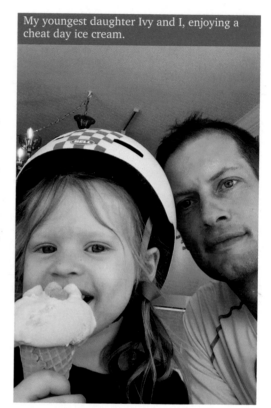

My youngest daughter Ivy and I, enjoying a cheat day ice cream.

• Leading brand cookies have 14-16 grams
• Ketchup serving more than 4 grams
• Pasta sauce has 16 grams
• Leading salad dressing has 3 to 5 grams
• One can of soda has 39 grams

Aside from our everyday food consumption, cultural celebrations also strongly influence our relationship with food. Although it may seem innocuous, all you have to do is pick any holiday or a celebratory occasion and you will likely be relating it to some form of sweet indulgence. To no surprise, Halloween tops the charts as the number one candy-selling holiday in the United States. For

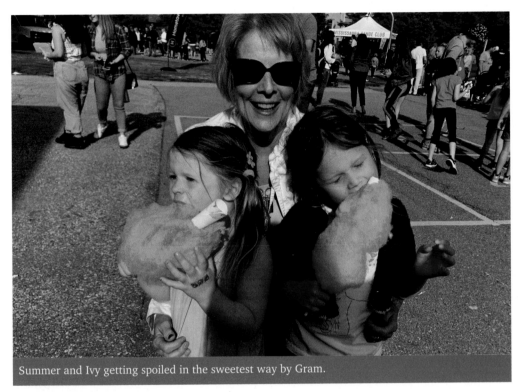
Summer and Ivy getting spoiled in the sweetest way by Gram.

that special day, over 600 million pounds of candy are sold yearly, equating to 2.75 billion dollars. The next contenders are Easter (65 million pounds sold) and Valentine's Day (48 million pounds of candy sold).[67]

The point is that culturally, we are continually exposing our children to large amounts of sugar, which normalizes the consumption and also makes it really tough for them to resist. And much like adults, the more children eat refined sugar, the more they will crave it and in higher quantities, filling themselves up with sugary foods instead of nutrient-filled ones. Much like us adults, their bodies aren't made to process such high sugar intake.

What does consuming more than the daily recommended amount of processed sugar on regular basis actually do to kids? There is evidence to suggest that hyperactivity and subsequent crashes happen, making it harder for them to concentrate and learn in a traditional school setting.[68] The long-term side effects are much worse: A higher risk of insulin resistance, prediabetes, Type 2 diabetes, Obesity and more.[69] Recent research has gone so far as to link today's obesity epidemic with childhood sugar intake decades ago.[70]

Dr. David S. Ludwig, director of the obesity program at Children's Hospital in Boston predicts that due to rising obesity rates and associated illnesses, our children's generation "could be the first in the history of the United States to live less healthy and shorter lives than their parents."[71]

What can we personally do to set ourselves and our children up for a healthier outlook? One tip from our house is that we let the girls pick 10 treats after Halloween. Shortly thereafter, the "candy fairy" arrives and in exchange for candy they get a surprise in the form of an experience like a visit to their favorite park or coloring books, markers, crafts, etc.

Aside from that, here are a few of my other favorites on how to approach the topic of sugar with our younger generation and empower them to make healthier choices.

5 Ways to Set Kids Up for Success!
No one wants to intentionally fail and most of us, including our kids, don't want to be constantly preached to about what is good for us. So here are a few tips on how to encourage kids to eat healthy, nutritious, no added sugar foods.

1. Create a Healthy Environment
You wouldn't expect someone who lived in a candy shop to never sample the sweets, would you? It may seem blatantly obvious, but if you want your kids to make this change with you, a solid start is to surround them with healthy options. You can't teach them about the perils of added sugar while having a fridge full of soda, a freezer full of ice cream, or cupboards full of cookies and candies. Temptation is much harder if not impossible to resist if the junk food is easily accessible. Ensure that healthy options are the prevalent ones in your house.

Retail psychologists have mastered product placement within stores, placing the items they want us to buy at our eye level, end caps (at the end of the aisle) and around the cash. Products that are placed in those locations often get included as spontaneous reach purchase.

Why not try to do the same at home? Place healthy snack options within their reach or at eye-level. Try cutting up fruit or veggie sticks and leave them in their play area or by their computer.

Another quick tip that we do in our home is to designate a snack area of healthy options in the fridge or in the pantry that kids are allowed to eat at any time of day. For a fridge area, think precut fruit, veggies, hummus, plain yogurts, nuts, seeds, nut butters (if there are no allergies), cheese strings or cubes, and hard boiled eggs. Good options for snack drawers include popcorn, nori /seaweed sheets, unsweetened dried fruit like figs or raisins or No Sugar Co snacks. Some of the kid's products that we have in the works are mentioned in the next chapter.

2. Eat and Experiment Together
Research shows that families that eat together at least once a day, consume more

fruits and vegetables and less fast food and sugary beverages.[72] Kids are indeed like sponges. They watch what we do. They emulate what they see. They want to follow the same paths we take. Eating together ensures that they have a good example to follow. So again, it may be obvious, but do your best to set a regular eating schedule and have at least one meal a day as a family, screen-free. One thing we've been doing for years is asking the same question: "What was the best part of your day?" and we all share. It's so simple yet such a great way to share details about our lives. Share the time to speak about the day and eat food mindfully. If television is currently present during mealtime, you may meet strong opposition initially as kids will not be happy about eating screen-free, but know that the battle will be worth it. Try to ease them into it or reserve it for a movie night after dinner. Eating while distracted by digital means such as phones or televisions, results in a higher consumption of calories. Mindless eating simply means eating more and often leads to overeating.[73]

You can also try cooking with your kids, always using that experience as a means to introduce new foods to their diets. This will broaden their diets and knowledge and condition them to be open minded about eating healthier fare.

When it comes to picky eaters, if you offer a healthy side or two, we found that a rule of "try it before refusing" tends to work. Surprisingly, it seems that children may need as many as 15 exposures to a new food before they finally accept it![74] In the famous words of Dr. Suess "try it, try it and you may, try it and you may I say (like it)". Eating with your family and making the family dinner a part of your regular routine is a great way to bring your family together and help your kids eat healthier.

3. Empower Children
I see a great sense of pride in my girls when they are able to make their own choices and be involved. Try to present them with a few healthy options and let them choose whenever possible. It could be as simple as deciding what ingredients they want to put in their smoothie, or what to top their plain oatmeal or unsweetened yogurt with. Just make sure that they are choosing from healthy options.

Also, getting them involved in cooking is a great way to teach them a life skill, spend some time with them, and empower them to contribute. Get them to choose a recipe, learn about ingredients and measurements (one of the sneaky added benefits of baking is learning math and fractions). Yes, mess is inevitable, but it is very common that a child will feel a sense of ownership and be willing to eat the food they helped prepare.

4. Make Food Interesting
In addition to the unspoken guidance mentioned above where planning and behavior modeling are important, there are also plenty of opportunities to have an open dialogue about food and sugar. In my opinion, these conversations should be positive and intentional, positioning food as the fuel for our body and something we enjoy, rather

than restrict and fear. Teach your kids about where food comes from. Take them to a farm and show them vegetables growing from the earth and fruits hanging from trees. Make it an experience and they will thirst for more.

As another example, take them to your yard and teach them about how plants get their colors, taste, and aroma from compounds called phytochemicals. Generally speaking, different colors are indicative of nutritional components that the fruit or vegetable may have. For example, green plants that are considered to be the healthiest of the bunch are high in vitamins K, B, and E, all of which are great for regulating blood sugars, lowering cholesterol, cardiovascular, and bone health.[75] As far as kids are concerned, they may be happy just hearing that green foods are good for their muscles, orange for their eyes, red for heart, yellow for speed, and blue for their growth. As a general rule of thumb, the more varied the colors of foods are on our plate, the higher the chances are that you're getting the necessary daily nutrient intake. Buy the (real food) rainbow and eat the rainbow. Try making some fruit kabobs or, take a page from my wife's playbook and make smiley faces on your kid's plates using cookie cutter shapes out of cucumber or watermelon.

5. Words Matter

How we talk about food with our kids matters. Food should be positioned as a nourishment for our bodies versus something that needs to restricted, feared, or controlled. I admit, even I have given in to an occasional ice cream request at the end of a long hike. Grandparents, I'm also looking at you here—I know when you sneak in the donuts! My personal take is that no matter how bad sugar may be for them, it isn't something that should be feared or demonized. Even if a child may be overweight, at the end of the day, they are still kids and don't need the extra stress. We can help them if we reduce their access to sugar, make it less frequent, make the portions smaller, present them with healthier options and let them be kids. I believe that occasional indulgence should be allowed.

It does help if the expectations are set ahead of time on when they can have that dessert. This way, if they ask for it frequently, your answer can be "I'm sorry, it's not in the plans for today. We will have it on the weekend." For those who have competitive spirit going, challenge your family to have at least one "no sugar day" each week and turn it into a game. It works well to set the expectations for everyone involved.

What I am not on board with is using foods for incentives, rewards, or punishments. The reason for this is that it's very easy for children to associate their successes, or failures and frustration with food. Fallen off a bike? Failed that exam? Sorry, a sugary snack unfortunately isn't the answer. If the habit is set early, it's likely to continue without intentional intervention into adulthood.

In our home, food is for nourishment. We

Remember to Hydrate

This may seem like another obvious piece of advice but it's important that children are able to stay hydrated primarily through plain water. Most of us by now have heard about the dangers of pop or soda. Fruit juices may sound like a good idea given that they are derived from fruit. However, they contain calories and added sugar, while the necessary nutrients like fiber are stripped away. Some dietitians claim that giving kids juice is nearly as bad as pop, as the combination of acid and sugar within them can cause significant tooth decay.[76] Make it easy on yourself and offer plain water, or if you want to make it fancy, occasional unflavored soda water. We often squirt in fresh lemon, lime, or grapefruit to make tastier sparkling water taste better.

---

don't reward with calories. Achievements are rewarded by offering experiences like a movie night, crafts, or playing their favorite game.

Parties

Let's face it: You can't control every meal your kids will eat. From school lunches and friends' birthday parties to going to a restaurant with you or attending events, what your kids eat is often out of your control. That's why it's so important to make sure they understand this lifestyle and the value of eating healthier food. With that foundation of healthy eating habits that you helped build, they will be able to make their own choices and select the best options available.

With that in mind, here are some quick tips to give to your kids for these situations:

Eating at a restaurant: Your kids will already know that veggies are a big part of any healthy meal, so they'll look for salads and healthier sides, but make sure they know it's OK to ask for dressings on the side. Kids may not think it's alright to ask for substitutions, but they need to know that they can ask their server for what they want to eat if they don't see it on the menu.

Visiting a friend's house: Whether it's a sleepover, play date, or study session that becomes staying over for dinner, it can be awkward to turn down snacks or meals at a friend's house. First and foremost, teach your kids that it is totally OK to politely refuse something they are offered. My girls, for example, don't like whipped cream so I've seen them turn down the offer nicely or allow just a taste to sample it, which is a great way to appease the host without having to eat something you don't really want. Attending an event: When did an event become so inherently tied to eating? An event should be just that: An event. My girls don't go to a sporting event, movie, or family gathering anticipating food. Instead, we talk about what they will do and the people they will get to have fun with.

However, it can be hard to dodge all the food in these scenarios so try to ensure

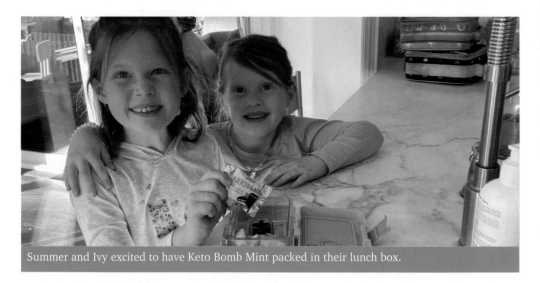

Summer and Ivy excited to have Keto Bomb Mint packed in their lunch box.

they don't leave home hungry. But while at the event, we take the relaxed approach and allow them to make their own food choices.

School lunches: If you're finding packing school lunches stressful, you are not alone! We have picky eaters, too, who regularly make requests for items that they've seen in their friend's lunch boxes. We do throw in an occasional indulgent treat but make our best attempt to include a balanced meal with fruit, veggies, carbs, and lean protein. We often give them a choice between an item or two, so they feel empowered and have a sense of ownership, which makes it more likely that they will eat the food.

Final Thoughts

There's a lot of great information out there about how to talk to your kids about any subject. While this book offers a few tips, what I want to highlight most is that you actually do talk to your kids about food and the role it plays in their lives. Millions of very young children have no concept of what health even means or where their food comes from. Yet, they spend their entire young lives consuming media that is targeting them and making them want snacks, drinks, burgers, and so much more, and connecting those things to an exciting life. The onus is on us, the parents, the caregivers, and the community to cut through the marketing and teach our kids what truly matters.

I feel so passionate about this that No Sugar Co. is investing into an entire product line of healthier alternatives for children that includes kids' bars, cookies, gummies and more! The premium ingredients for these products cost much more than what's currently being put into many of their comparative snacks. I am consciously making the decision knowing that we will be losing money on most of the kids snacks sales in the first little while but I am hopeful that we will find a way to eventually produce the treats on a larger scale and at a more efficient cost.

That's how we wholeheartedly believe in this investment and in providing our children with snacks that don't contain processed sugar.

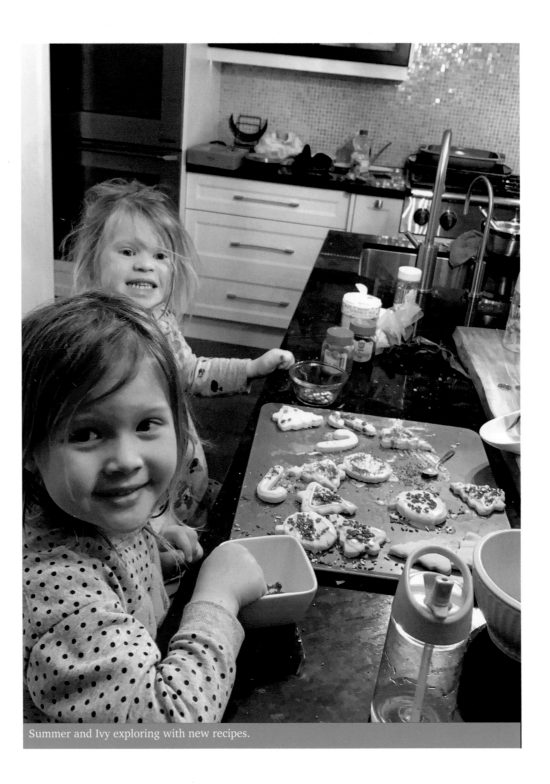

Summer and Ivy exploring with new recipes.

Chapter 08

LOOKING FORWARD WITH NO SUGAR COMPANY

Ingredients that don't help to improve the health of those who eat them. While that may seem like a simple venture, it takes a lot of work to get even one product off the ground and into consumers' hands. This chapter will look at what we do behind closed doors, but more importantly our future plans, and how we want to grow with you.

What Matters Most: Our Ingredients
When I decided to launch the No Sugar Company, I made it a part of our corporate promise that we would not be using added sugars to make our products taste good. That is our core principle, but what's inside each product we make is much more than just a no-sugar-added food. I wanted to make each product healthy as well. That meant redefining how these sorts of

packaged foods were made. The result was that the No Sugar Company had to deliver on more than one promise, so we distilled that to four rules that guide everything we produce.

Our Four Guiding Principles
• No Sugar: Provide healthier alternatives to our favorite products.
• Great Taste: Dedicated to melt-in your mouth flavor with no sacrifice in taste in lieu of sugar.
• High Quality Ingredients: No compromises, the best, clean, ingredients we can source.
• Better Choices: For ourselves, our loved ones and our communities.

With these principles as our North star, we moved fast into trying to find ingredients that would make our products the very best in class.

Processed sugar and fillers are cheap. What we use isn't.

As we've covered throughout this book, we rely on stevia and/or erythritol to make our products sweet without empty calories and processed sugar. In terms of cost, Stevia is about 72 times more expensive than refined sugar. In addition to that, we use custom-made, responsibly-sourced dark chocolate, high-quality proteins, only the best and ethically sourced, healthiest of fats like premium coconut oil and nut butters. All of this makes our food NON-GMO, keto-friendly, and gluten-free, with no added sugars, additives, or fillers—just good, healthy, delicious food.

Research, Development, and Delivery
Any new product in any industry must start with the consumer. With that in mind, everything we create at the No Sugar Co is based exclusively on the data we get on what consumers are looking for combined with our collective marketplace knowledge. From there, we formulate an idea for a product creating something as special as our No Sugar Keto Cups/Bombs.

We already know that the world of nutrition is drastically changing. After years of being inundated with high sugar, high carb foods, consumers are ready for healthier alternatives, which is at the forefront of everything we make at the No Sugar Co. Working within the rules listed above, we try to source the best ingredients necessary to make a new product. Usually that means sourcing new ingredients that work with those that we know deliver the goods. Then we test. And we test. And we test. And we test. It's not uncommon for a new product to go through dozens of versions—frequently more than 100 versions—before we create something that we are happy with. And we don't stop there because we're always trying to evolve, tweak, and improve our products.

When a formula, or prototype, is created, we then must ensure that the product has shelf stability and can sustain being packaged, shipped, delivered, and sold while still tasting great when it is in your hands and you're ready to eat. That's another process that takes a great number of iterations, tests, and refinements to reach success. It's also why all of our food has relatively short shelf-life compared to the competition and on some of them, a call to refrigerate. Synthetic 'food' might promise to last nearly forever, but real food like what we create does not.

No Sugar Is For Everyone!
I frequently get asked who should eat our products and my answer is: Everyone! Although our products have no refined sugar, they don't compromise on taste, so they are a nutritious and tasty snack for all. They are also diabetic friendly, those who are on low-carb or keto diet, those who avoid gluten, and are excellent snacks for children. Some of our products are also dairy free.

No Sugar Company & Kids

Like I said previously, the health of my two daughters is of utmost importance to me, which is the driving force behind some of our upcoming products. After much product development and testing, we've chosen their favorite flavors, and even named the bars after them. But to be honest, when it comes to snacks, the kid's category is one of the most difficult ones to succeed in on a global level. The reality is that most children don't care about how healthy a product is or even how much you paid for it. They judge the snack on its taste and texture, and ultimately its sweetness level, too. The majority of the products that are launched in the kid's snack category fail. Why? Because the majority of healthier versions of their favorite foods without sugar simply don't taste good enough to them, given that their taste buds are expecting sugar.

As high as that risk of entering the kid's category may be, I am willing to take it as I wholeheartedly believe that we should be offering our future generations healthier alternatives with no refined sugars. As such, we will soon be launching an entire line of kids' snacks including No Sugar Kids bars, No Sugar Kids Gummies, and No Sugar Kids cookies, with more to come. Our mission is to create products that taste amazing and that kids love, and that also have ingredients that parents feel good about.

On that note, I am inviting you to come along for the journey and if you do decide to give these products a try as they become available, please share your honest feedback and thoughts with us. I really want to get this right and change kid's nutrition for good!

On a more personal note, we have chosen to build a Be Brave. Be Yourself.TM no-bullying campaign. This is very near and dear to my heart as my wife Mel, who grew up in a small Canadian town, had terrible bullying experiences growing up. You can read some of the stories she felt comfortable sharing to better understand why this mission is so important to us in the 'Note on Our Mission from Mel.' We want to ensure that all of our children have the proper education and resources to cope should they find themselves in that unfortunate situation. In each box of our No Sugar Kids bars, we will include bracelets to empower children and remind them to Be Brave, Be YourselfTM and to stand up for themselves and others. Proceeds of each sale will also be shared amongst like-minded charities that support the cause of confidence building and no-bullying.

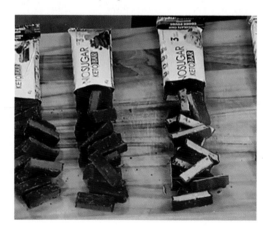

A Note on our Family Mission from Mel Woodgate

Being bullied in both elementary and high school was one of the hardest things that I went through growing up. There was no awareness or education or resources to turn to for students, educators, or parents. I was very fortunate to have a very loving and supportive family but even then, I did not tell my parents or sister everything that was happening at school. I grew up in Thunder Bay, Ontario, Canada, where small class sizes were common and unless someone moved into or out of your neighborhood, you were with the same kids throughout most of your school years.

In elementary school, I remember being ignored by all the girls in class because the bully told them they would have to pay a dollar to her if they talked to me. I was left mean notes in my desk regularly and probably the worst experience was when I was in grade 5 and I walked into class and saw all the girls wearing a pin on their shirts that had my class picture on it and the devil drawn around my face with 666 written under it.

In high school, I was left out of parties, had notes left on my locker, and rumors spread about me that weren't true. Maya Angelou has said it best: "you may not remember what some said, or what someone did, but you will always remember how it made you feel."

Fast forward 30 years to today where there is so much more awareness centered around bullying from Pink T-shirt day, to hotlines, and 24hr support, as well as resources for parents and educators. This is all great and it has come so far, but I know there is still work to be done. I am determined to make a change not only because I have two daughters but because of what I went through and what so many other kids still go through today. It is so important to teach kids to Be Brave and to Be Yourself and not let their self-worth be decided by the outside world like I did. I am so excited to see the positive impact the No Sugar Kids Bar will have on our mission to our no bullying efforts.

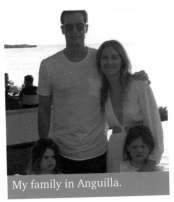

My family in Anguilla.

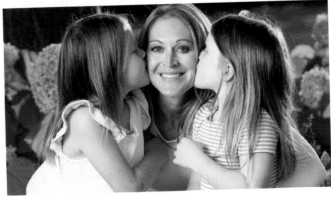

Building A Community

My dream for the No Sugar Company is to become a true disruptor in the food industry and beyond, changing the way we approach our relationship with food and also in the ways that we connect and support one another in the effort to lead a healthier life. I invite you to be a part of our No Sugar community!

Tell us about your struggles and triumphs, which products you would like to see in the market, and how we can jointly make this no sugar movement a healthier, happier journey for you.

Share your thoughts with us @nosugarcompany or with me personally @nosugarco.ceo. And once our free No Sugar In Me app is live, let's connect with one another there and Crush Your Sugar Cravings, one craving at a time!

I hope that I have given you some food for thought in these pages and some motivation to lead a healthier life by saying No Sugar in Me. With that, I thank you for taking the time to read this and wish you the sweetest of successes in your personal no sugar journey!

The No Sugar Revolution is here, and with this book and the No Sugar Company by your side for support, you're leading the way!

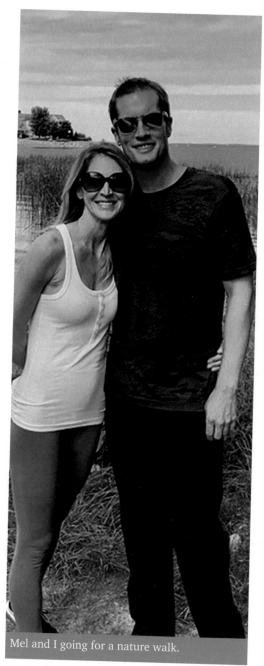

Mel and I going for a nature walk.

I want to hear how your experience with No Sugar In Me is going!

Let me know how you are progressing in your personal No Sugar journey and if you have any feedback on what you've learned in this book or on our products.

Find me on Instagram on **@nosugarco.ceo** and **@nosugarcompany** or visit us at **thenosugarcompany.com** to shop our No Sugar Company products and earn some sweet No Sugar Rewards.

Thank you for taking the time to read this and for taking on refined sugar.

Your body will thank you!

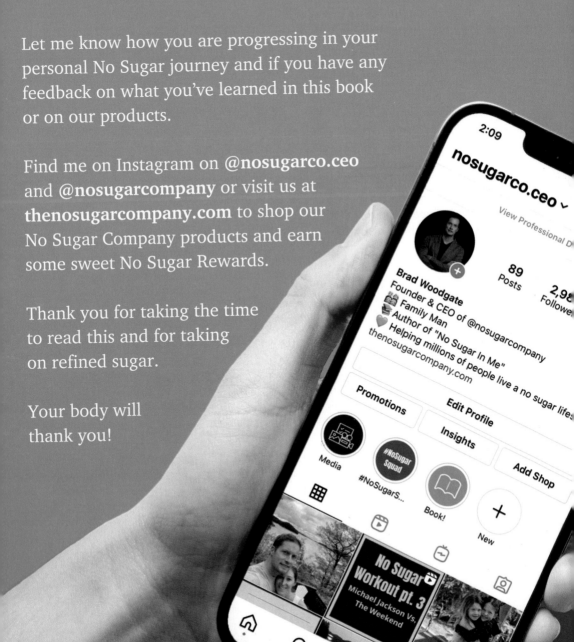

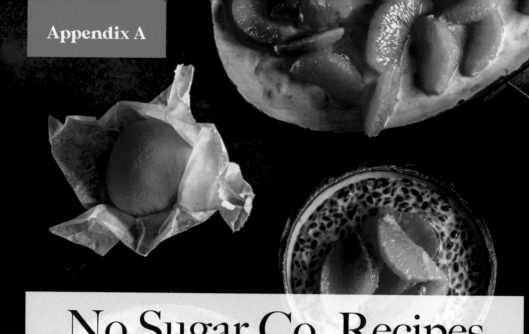

No Sugar Co. Recipes

As an added bonus, I also wanted to provide you with a few recipe options to inspire you. They are wonderful if you're entertaining, celebrating a special occasion or are just looking to add a boost to your daily meals. I intentionally chose recipes that may not be in your everyday cooking repertoire but are still relatively easy to whip up and are amazingly tasty with no to low sugar. If you're adhering to a specialty diet, feel free to substitute with appropriate alternatives and really make them your own. So browse, explore and enjoy!

LEGEND

GF - Gluten Free   K - Keto   VG - Vegetarian

BREAKFAST

Fancy Toast

Green Glow Smoothie GF-VG

Power Oatmeal Bowl VG

Keto Pancakes GF-K-VG

Dutch Baby Pancakes GF-K-VG

Keto Granola GF-K-VG

LUNCH

Beetroot Carpaccio Salad GF-K

Peas in a Pod Soup GF-K-VG

Quick Lettuce Wraps GF-K

Smoked Salmon Crostini K

Energy Boost Salad GF

Mason Jar Salad GF-K

Keto Tomato Soup GF-K-VG

Chicken Salad With
Avocado Salsa GF-K

Cauliflower Pizza GF

APPETIZERS

Tuna Tartare GF-K

Baked Brie GF-K-VG

Smoked Salmon Rolls GF-K

Guacamole with Bacon Chips GF-K

DINNER

Basil Pesto Pasta VG

Salmon Steak GF-K

Summer Scallops GF-K

Roasted Chicken GF-K

Mussels Fra Diavolo GF-K

Keto Alfredo Pasta GF-K

Keto Lasagna GF-K-VG

Crispy Pork Belly GF-K-VG

Cordon Bleu GF-K-VG

Stuffed Red Pepper GF-K

DESSERTS

Keto Chocolate Milk GF-K

Keto Chocolove Muffins K-VG

Stellar Chia Pudding GF-K-VG

Frosty Chocolate
Keto Shake GF-K-VG

Keto Bomb Brownies GF-K-VG

Keto Lemon Bars GF-K-VG

BREAKFAST

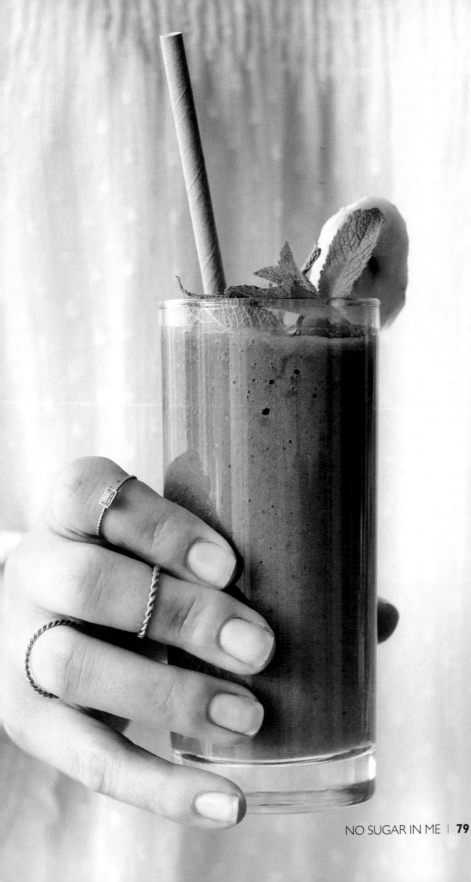

Fancy Toast

Prep Time: 10 minutes | Cook Time: 5 minutes | Total Time: 15 minutes

1 Serving

Ingredients

- Whole grain bread
- Half of avocado
- Hummus
- Two eggs
- Beet sprouts
- Black sesame seeds
- Some butter

Method

1. Roast 2 slices of wholegrain bread in a skillet until nice and crispy.
2. Fry eggs with some butter in a pan within a large cookie cutter, so they keep a tight shape, season and place them on the first slice of toast.
3. Add some hummus on second slice and add your thinly sliced avocado.
4. Garnish with some beet sprouts and sesame seeds.

NUTRITION FACTS

SERVINGS: 1

amount per serving			DV%			DV%
CALORIES **462**	Total Fat	33.7 g	43%	Total Carbohydrates	25.6 g	9%
	Saturated Fat	7.7 g	39%	Dietary Fiber	10.2 g	36%
NET CARBS **15.4 g**	Cholesterol	327 mg	109%	Total Sugars	2 g	
	Sodium	441 mg	19%	Protein	18.3 g	

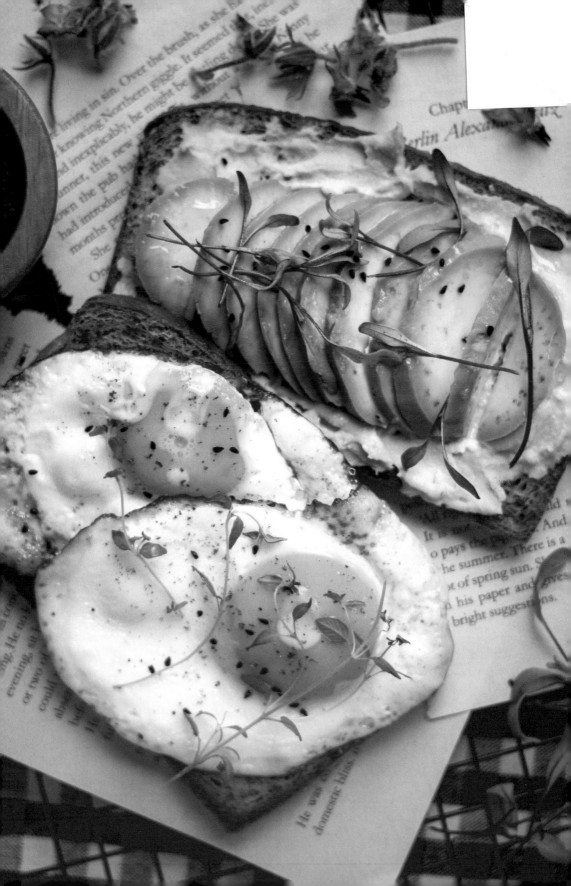

Green Glow Smoothie

Prep Time: 10 minutes | *Cook Time: 0 minutes* | *Total Time: 10 minutes*

2 Servings
GF-VG

Ingredients

- 2 cups fresh pineapple
- 4 cups fresh spinach
- 2 medium bananas
- 1 cup of peeled apples

Method

1. Add pineapples, spinach, bananas and apples to a blender. Blend it all together until smooth, pausing to scrape down the sides if needed.

2. Serve and enjoy! This smoothie will last in your fridge for up to 2 days.

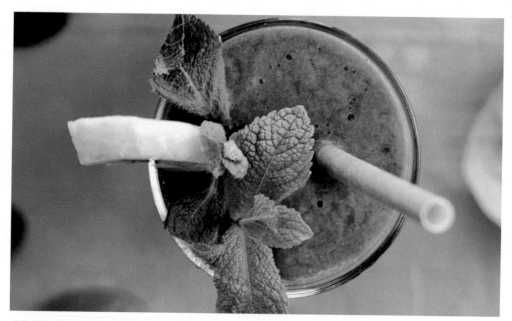

NUTRITION FACTS

SERVINGS: 2

amount per serving			DV%			DV%
CALORIES **257**	Total Fat	1.1 g	1%	Total Carbohydrates	63.7 g	23%
	Saturated Fat	0.2 g	1%	Dietary Fiber	6.9 g	25%
NET CARBS **56.8 g**	Cholesterol	0 mg	0%	Total Sugars	41.3 g	
	Sodium	52 mg	2%	Protein	4.8 g	

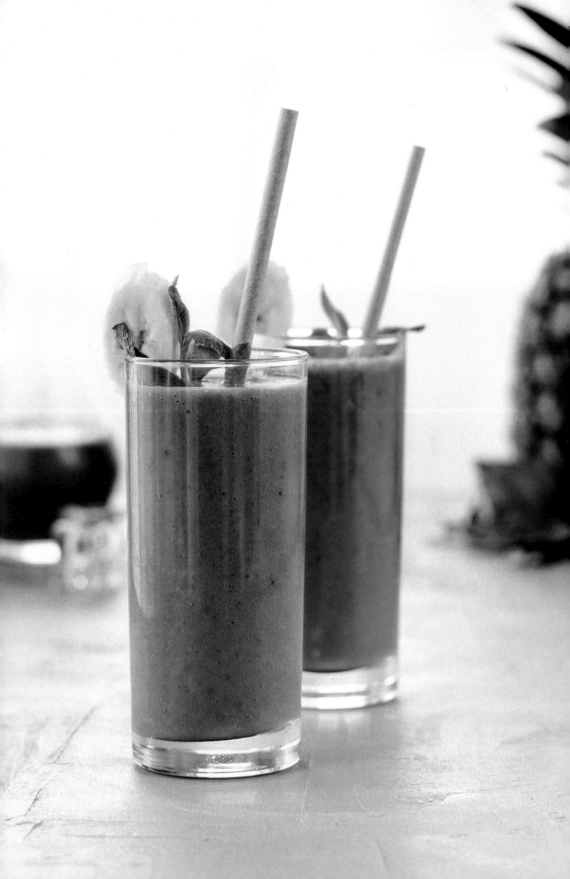

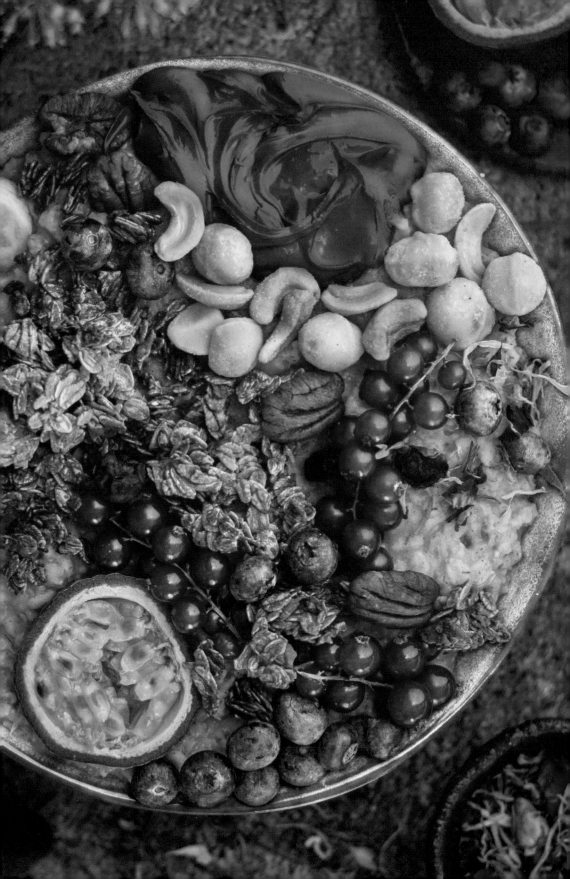

Power Oatmeal Bowl

Prep Time: 10 minutes | Cook Time: 15 minutes | Total Time: 25 minutes

2 Servings
VG

Ingredients

- 3.5 oz oats
- 1 cup milk of choice
- 1 tsp cinnamon
- 1 pinch of salt
- 1 tbsp Stevia
- 1 tbsp vanilla protein powder (optional)
- Toppings of your choice can include some nuts, blueberries, red currant and granola and some melted or crushed No Sugar Co. Keto Krax

METHOD

Add all ingredients for oatmeal to a saucepan (except protein powder). Bring to the boil, reduce heat to medium and simmer for 5 minutes until creamy. Stir regularly. Set aside for 2 minutes to cool down a little bit. Stir in the protein powder, top with your favorite toppings and you are ready to go!

No Sugar Co. Keto Krax makes a great topping!

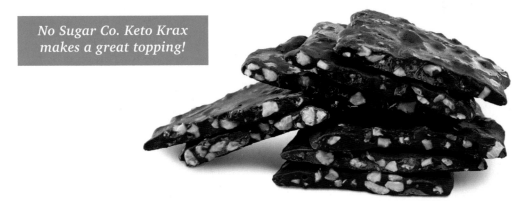

NUTRITION FACTS

SERVINGS: 2

amount per serving			DV%			DV%
CALORIES **249**	Total Fat	5.7 g	7%	Total Carbohydrates	39.6 g	14%
	Saturated Fat	2.1 g	10%	Dietary Fiber	5 g	18%
NET CARBS **34.6 g**	Cholesterol	10 mg	3%	Total Sugars	6 g	
	Sodium	60 mg	3%	Protein	10.5 g	

Keto Pancakes

Prep Time: 15 minutes | Cook Time: 10 minutes | Total Time: 25 minutes

12 Pieces

GF-K-VG

Ingredients

- 1 cup Almond flour
- 1/4 cup Coconut flour
- 2-3 tbsp Erythritol
- 1 tsp Baking powder
- 5 large Eggs
- 1/3 cup Unsweetened Almond milk
- 1/4 cup Avocado oil
- 1 1/2 tsp Vanilla extract
- 1/4 tsp Sea salt
- Melted No Sugar Keto Cups of your choice
- Strawberries

Method

1. In a bowl, combine all ingredients and whisk until smooth. The batter should have a typical pancake consistency.

2. Add some avocado oil to a nonstick pan, and over medium heat, drop the batter into the hot pan, forming small circles.

3. Cook for around 2 minutes, or until you see bubbles start to form.

4. Flip and cook covered for another 2 minutes, or until nicely browned

5. Melt some No Sugar Keto cups of your choice and pour over your finished pancakes, garnish with strawberries.

NUTRITION FACTS (SAUCE ONLY)

SERVINGS: 4

amount per serving			DV%			DV%
CALORIES **181**	Total Fat	11.5 g	15%	Total Carbohydrates	10.4 g	4%
	Saturated Fat	2.9 g	14%	Dietary Fiber	5.2 g	18%
NET CARBS **5.2 g**	Cholesterol	205 mg	68%	Total Sugars	1.9 g	
	Sodium	80 mg	3%	Protein	9.9 g	

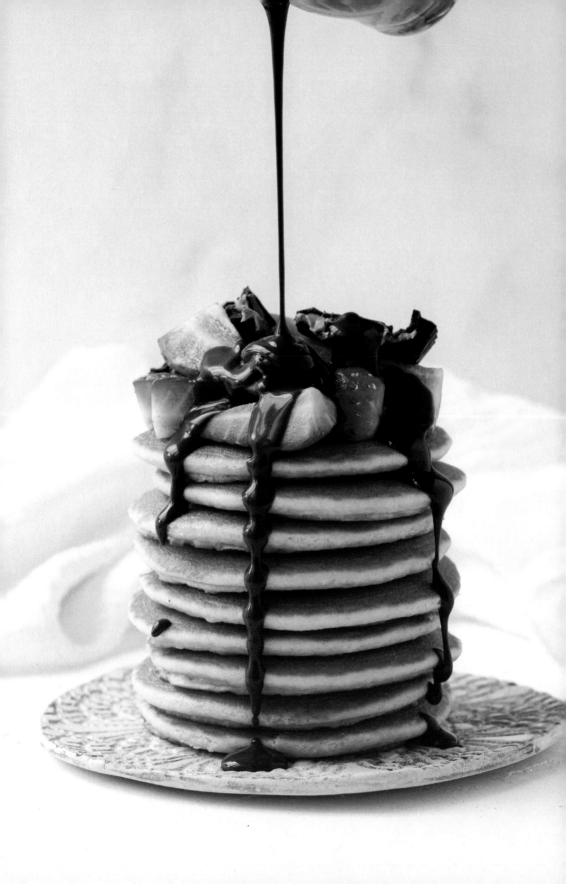

Dutch Baby Pancakes

Prep Time: 10 minutes | *Cook Time: 20 minutes* | *Total Time: 30 minutes*

4 Servings
GF-K-VG

Ingredients

- 3 large eggs
- 3 tbsp stevia, powdered
- 2/3 cup whole milk
- 2/3 cup all-purpose gluten-free flour
- 1½ tsp vanilla extract
- Salt
- Grated nutmeg
- 2 tbsp butter
- 2 cups berries of your choice

Method

1. You will need a 10-inch cast-iron pan.
2. Preheat the oven to 425ºF, and put your pan into the oven to heat it.
3. Beat the eggs and stevia with an electric hand mixer until light and frothy.
4. Add in the milk, flour, vanilla, salt and grated nutmeg, and beat until you have a smooth and thin batter.
5. Using an oven mitt, remove the pan from the oven and put the batter carefully into the hot pan.
6. Return immediately to the oven.
7. Bake until puffed and golden brown, around 20 minutes.
8. Dust with powdered stevia and top with fresh berries.

NUTRITION FACTS

SERVINGS: 4

amount per serving			DV%			DV%
CALORIES **237**	Total Fat	21 g	27%	Total Carbohydrates	7.5 g	3%
	Saturated Fat	3.82 g	19%	Dietary Fiber	4.9 g	17%
NET CARBS **2.6 g**	Cholesterol	10 mg	3%	Total Sugars	1.4 g	
	Sodium	32 mg	1%	Protein	7.2 g	

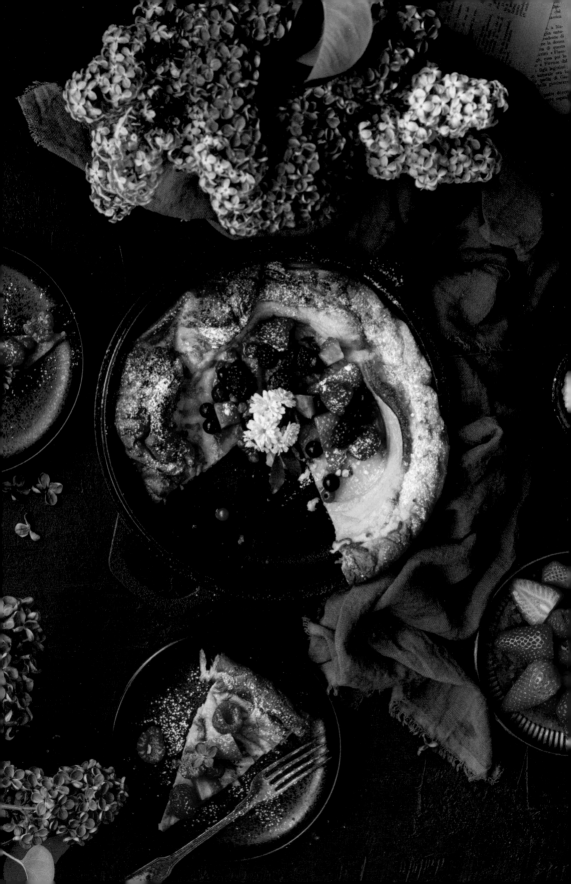

Keto Granola

Prep Time: 10 minutes | Cook Time: 15 minutes | Total Time: 25 minutes

12 Servings
GF-K-VG

Ingredients

- 1 cup Almonds
- 1 cup Hazelnuts
- 1 cup Pecans
- 1/3 cup Pumpkin seeds
- 1/3 cup Sunflower seeds
- 6 tbsp Erythritol
- 1/2 cup golden flaxseed meal
- 1 Egg white
- 1/4 cup butter, melted
- 1 tsp Vanilla extract

TOPPINGS

- 4 tbsp pomegranate
- 4 No Sugar Company Keto Cups
- 4 tbsp peanut butter

Method

1. Preheat your oven to 325°F and line a baking sheet with parchment paper.

2. In a food processor, roughly blitz almonds and hazelnuts, then add the pecans and pulse again. You want the nuts to be quartered, not too fine.

3. Add the pumpkin seeds, sunflower seeds, erythritol, and golden flaxseed meal. Pulse just until everything is combined.

4. Combine the vanilla, butter and egg white, add pulse a couple of times until everything is evenly coated, don't over-process.

5. Transfer the nut mixture to the prepared baking sheet, form into a tight rectangle and bake for 15 minutes, until lightly browned.

6. Cool completely before breaking into pieces. Serve with some greek yogurt, peanut butter, pomegranate and chopped No Sugar Keto Cups.

NUTRITION FACTS

SERVINGS: 12

amount per serving			DV%			DV%
CALORIES **237**	Total Fat	4.1 g	5%	Total Carbohydrates	34.7 g	13%
	Saturated Fat	1.2 g	6%	Dietary Fiber	1.7 g	6%
NET CARBS **33 g**	Cholesterol	140 mg	47%	Total Sugars	3.1 g	
	Sodium	93 mg	4%	Protein	9.1 g	

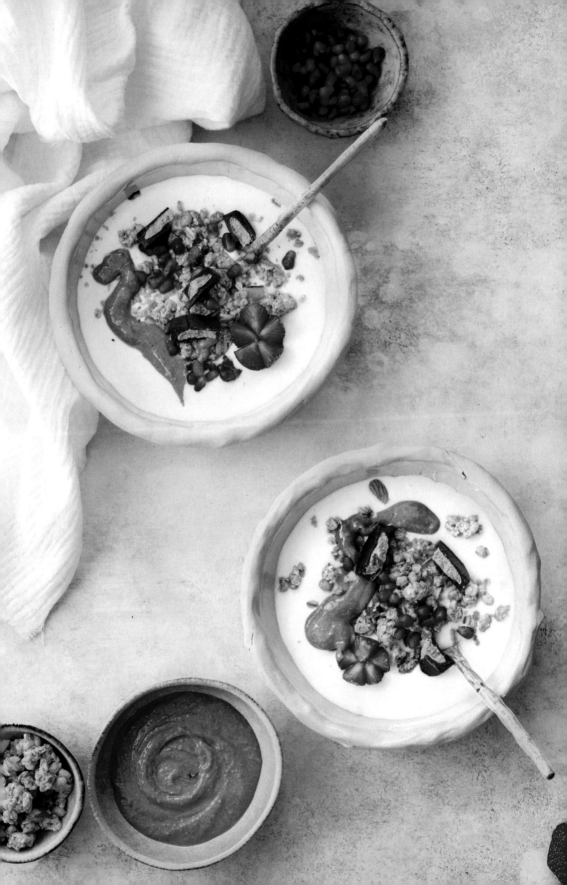

LUNCH

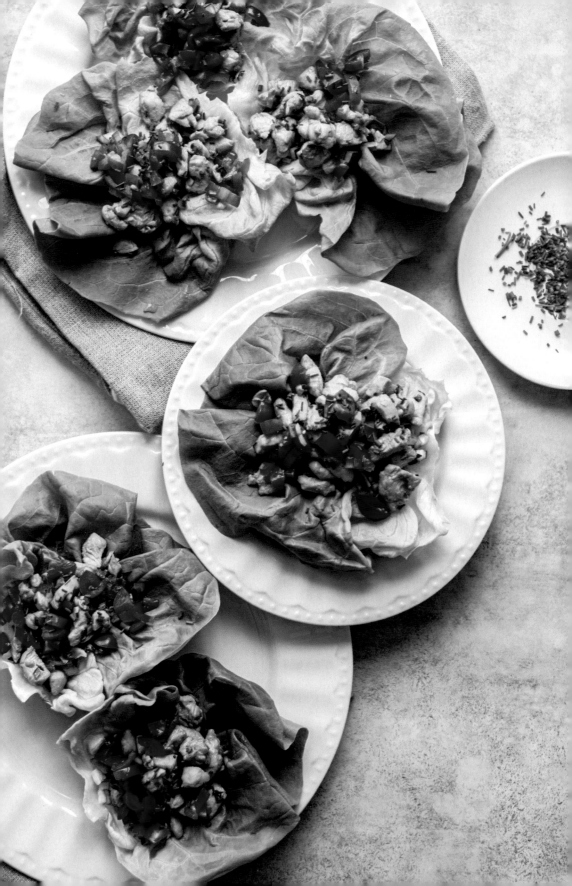

Beetroot Carpaccio Salad

Prep Time: 15 minutes | Cook Time: 60 minutes

2 Servings

GF-K

Ingredients

- 1 medium Beetroot
- ¼ cup walnuts
- Handful of rocket leaves
- 30g of feta

- Balsamic vinegar reduction
- ½ teaspoon of stevia
- Olive oil
- Salt and pepper
- Dill

Method

1. Pre-heat your oven to 180°F.
2. Wrap up your beetroot in tin foil and roast in the oven for 1 hour or until soft.
3. Remove the beetroot and place in a bowl of ice water to help peel off the skin.
4. Peel beetroot and chop off the ends.
5. With a mandoline slicer, carefully slice beetroot into thin circles and lay them down evenly on your plate.
6. To caramelize walnuts, place coconut oil, stevia and balsamic vinegar reduction in a pan and let it simmer.
7. Add walnuts and toss them in the mixture until coated and the liquid is starting to turn dark brown.
8. Place the rocket all over the dish and sprinkle over the feta cheese and caramelized walnuts.
9. Top with some good olive oil, reduced balsamic vinegar and salt and pepper.
10. Garnish with some dill. Enjoy!

NUTRITION FACTS

SERVINGS: 2

amount per serving			DV%			DV%
CALORIES **357**	Total Fat	33.4 g	43%	Total Carbohydrates	11 g	4%
	Saturated Fat	5.8 g	29%	Dietary Fiber	1.1 g	4%
NET CARBS **9.9 g**	Cholesterol	13 mg	4%	Total Sugars	3.7 g	
	Sodium	168 mg	7%	Protein	7.4 g	

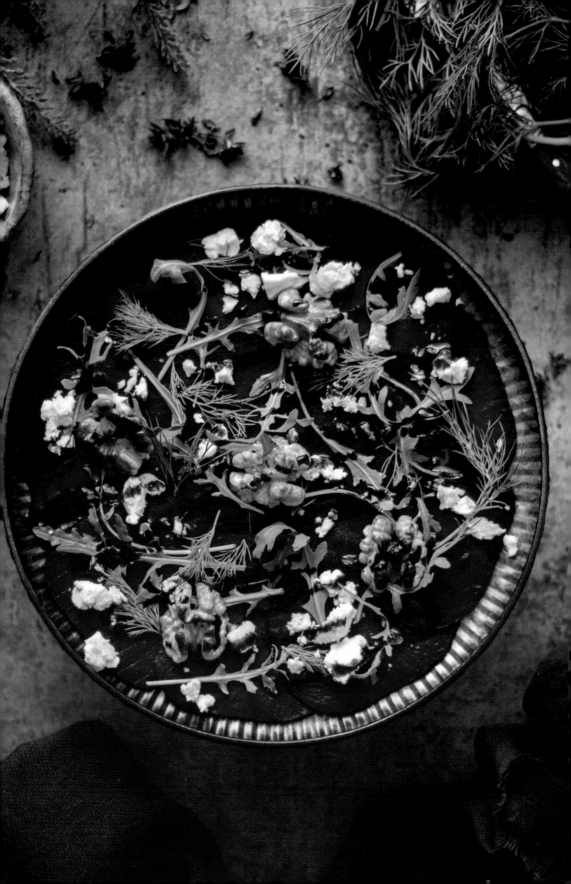

Peas in a Pod Soup

Prep Time: 5 minutes | Cook Time: 25 minutes | Total Time: 30 minutes

2 Servings
GF-K-VG

Ingredients

- 7 oz frozen peas
- 1 ¼ cups vegetable stock
- ¼ cup coconut cream
- 1 tbsp olive oil
- 1 garlic clove, chopped
- ½ onion, chopped
- Salt and freshly ground black pepper
- 2-3 mushrooms, sliced

METHOD

1. Heat the oil in a saucepan over medium heat. Add onion and garlic and fry for 3–4 minutes, until softened.

2. Add frozen peas and vegetable stock and bring to a boil. Reduce heat and simmer for ten minutes.

3. Add the coconut cream and use a hand blender to liquidize the soup.

4. In the meantime roast mushrooms on a lightly greased pan.

5. Season to taste and serve in a warm bowl (you can warm it up by running under hot water for one minute), garnished with some herbs, coconut cream and mushrooms.

NUTRITION FACTS

SERVINGS: 2

amount per serving			DV%			DV%
CALORIES **215**	Total Fat	14.5 g	19%	Total Carbohydrates	17.2 g	6%
	Saturated Fat	7.4 g	37%	Dietary Fiber	6.7 g	24%
NET CARBS' **10.5 g**	Cholesterol	0 mg	0%	Total Sugars	6.3 g	
	Sodium	126 mg	5%	Protein	6.3 g	

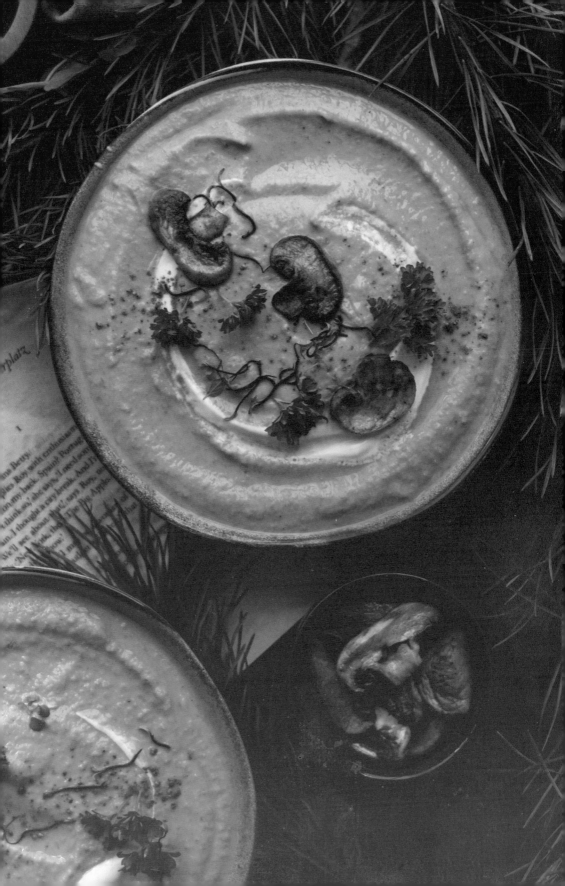

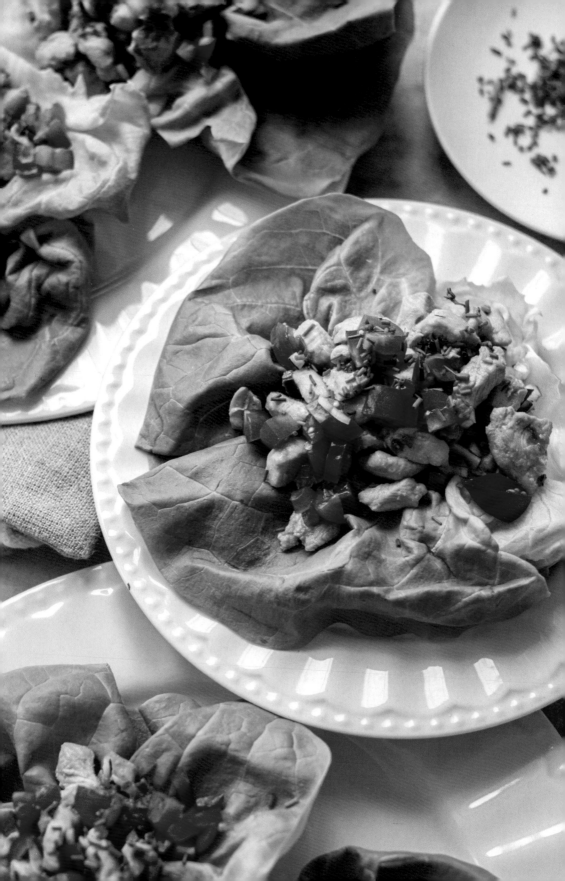

Quick Lettuce Wraps

Prep Time: 15 minutes | Cook Time: 15 minutes | Total Time: 30 minutes

4 Servings

GF-K

Ingredients

- 12-16 Bibb or butter lettuce leaves, washed and dried
- 1 pound chicken filets (or breast)
- 2 tablespoons olive oil
- 1 large red onion, chopped
- 4 cloves garlic, minced
- 3 tablespoons soy sauce
- 2 teaspoons fresh ginger, minced
- 10 cherry tomatoes, finely chopped
- 2 tablespoons chives, chopped

METHOD

1. Slice chicken into small cubes.
2. In a large skillet over medium-high heat, heat olive oil.
3. Add chicken, garlic, onions and fry for about 2-3 minutes, constantly stirring.
4. Once meat is well done add soy sauce, ginger and mix well. Turn off the heat and set aside.
5. Pack lettuce leaves with the filling, spoon over chopped tomatoes and sprinkle some fresh chives on top. Enjoy!

NOTE

Chicken can be substituted with your favorite ground meat.
Feel free to get creative and load it up with your favorite ingredients.

NUTRITION FACTS

amount per serving			DV%			DV%
CALORIES **257**	Total Fat	10.6 g	14%	Total Carbohydrates	14 g	5%
	Saturated Fat	1.1 g	6%	Dietary Fiber	4 g	14%
NET CARBS **10 g**	Cholesterol	73 mg	24%	Total Sugars	8.5 g	
	Sodium	750 mg	33%	Protein	27.7 g	

Smoked Salmon Crostini

Prep Time: 15 minutes | Cook Time: 10 minutes | Total Time: 25 minutes

8 Servings

K

Ingredients

- 6 oz | 170g goat cheese, at room temperature
- 3.5 oz | 100g smoked salmon
- 2 teaspoons lemon juice
- 2 tablespoons fresh thyme leaves, plus more for serving
- 1 loaf ciabatta bread, sliced

- Extra virgin olive oil, for drizzling
- Kosher salt and pepper
- 1/3 cup | 55g raspberries
- Basil pesto, for drizzling
- Some sage leaves
- Some pickled onion (optional

METHOD

1. Preheat your grill to high heat or preheat your oven to 400° F.

2. In a medium bowl, stir together goat cheese, lemon juice and thyme.

3. Place bread on a baking sheet and drizzle with olive oil on both sides of each slice, season with salt and pepper. Place the bread on the grill and grill both for about 2-3 minutes per side or until lightly toasted. Remove from the grill.

Spread goat cheese over bread and top with salmon, sliced beets, raspberries, some extra thyme and sage leaves. Season with salt and pepper. Top with pesto and pickled onions. Drizzle with olive oil. Serve and enjoy!

NUTRITION FACTS

SERVINGS: 8

amount per serving			DV%			DV%
CALORIES **345**	Total Fat	10.7 g	14%	Total Carbohydrates	50.3 g	5%
	Saturated Fat	5.6 g	28%	Dietary Fiber	3 g	7%
NET CARBS **11.5 g**	Cholesterol	25 mg	8%	Total Sugars	3.8 g	
	Sodium	704 mg	31%	Protein	15.9 g	

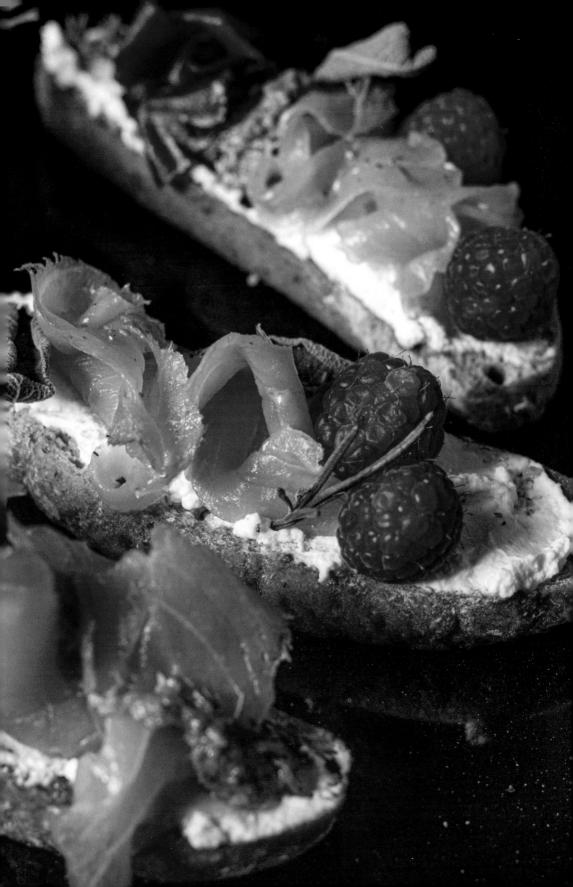

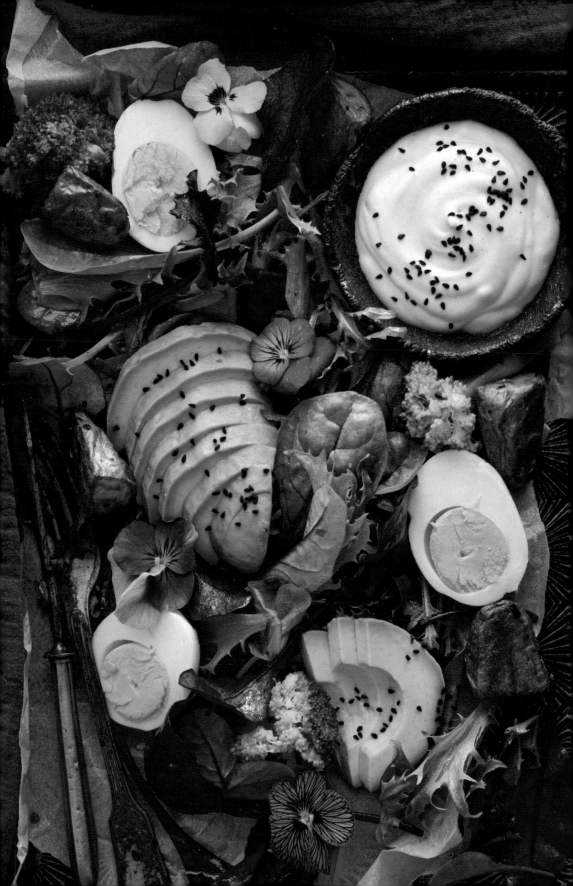

Energy Boost Salad

Prep Time: 15 minutes | *Cook Time: 30 minutes* | *Total Time: 50 minutes*

4 Servings
GF

Ingredients:

- 28 oz hard-boiled potatoes, quartered
- 2 whole avocados, sliced
- 7 oz broccoli florets
- 8 eggs, boiled
- 7 cups mixed salad greens
- 1 tsp black sesame seeds
- Homemade mayonnaise (optional)
- 7 tablespoons olive oil

Method

1. Preheat your oven to 400°F and place the potatoes on a baking tray.
2. Drizzle them with olive oil and sprinkle them with sea salt.
3. Roast for 30 minutes or until golden.
4. Boil the broccoli over medium-high heat until tender, rinse under cold water and set aside.
5. Add your salad mix to a bowl and drizzle with 7 tablespoons of olive oil. Mix well and arrange on a tray.
6. Top with broccoli, sliced avocados, baked potatoes and boiled eggs, as shown in the picture.
7. Serve with homemade mayonnaise. (optional)

NUTRITION FACTS

SERVINGS: 4

amount per serving			DV%			DV%
CALORIES **730**	Total Fat	55.8 g	71%	Total Carbohydrates	44.1 g	16%
	Saturated Fat	11.1 g	56%	Dietary Fiber	12.9 g	46%
NET CARBS **31.2 g**	Cholesterol	409 mg	136%	Total Sugars	4.5 g	
	Sodium	188 mg	8%	Protein	20.6 g	

Mason Jar Salad

Prep Time: 20 minutes | Cook Time: 5 minutes | Total Time: 26 minutes

2 Servings

GF-K

Ingredients For The Salad:

- 1/4 tsp sea salt
- 1/4 tsp garlic powder
- 1/8 tsp ground black pepper
- 1 tbsp extra virgin olive oil
- 2 chicken breasts, boneless and skinless
- 1 cucumber, peeled and sliced
- 1 cup cherry tomatoes, quartered
- 1 cup mixed salad greens
- 1/2 cup red onion, diced
- 1/2 cup carrot, grained

Ingredients For The DRESSING:

- 1/2 cup plain full-fat Greek yogurt
- 1/4 cup unsweetened almond milk
- 1 tbsp apple cider vinegar
- 1/4 tsp dill
- 1/4 tsp garlic powder
- 1/4 tsp sea salt

Method

1. Season the chicken breast with sea salt, black pepper, and garlic powder.
2. Heat olive oil in a skillet over medium-high heat.
3. Once hot, add the chicken and cook until well-browned on all sides and cooked through, about 4-6 minutes per side.
4. Dice into bite-size pieces and let cool.
5. For the dressing, whisk together all ingredients.
6. Using a 32 oz mason jar, layer about 2-4 tbsp. of the salad dressing, followed by the carrot, cucumber, cherry tomatoes, diced onion, chicken, and mixed salad greens.
7. Perfect for a summer picnic!

NUTRITION FACTS

SERVINGS: 2

amount per serving			DV%			DV%
CALORIES **275**	Total Fat	11.3 g	15%	Total Carbohydrates	13.5 g	5%
	Saturated Fat	1.7 g	9%	Dietary Fiber	2 g	7%
NET CARBS **11.5 g**	Cholesterol	75 mg	25%	Total Sugars	9.2 g	
	Sodium	130 mg	6%	Protein	29.1 g	

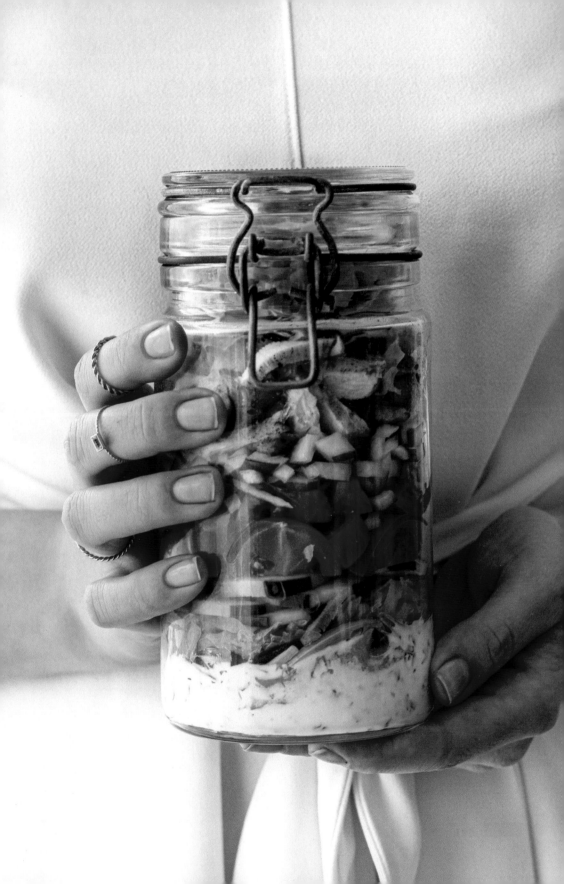

Keto Tomato Soup

Prep Time: 10 minutes | *Cook Time: 10 minutes* | *Total Time: 20 minutes*

4 Servings

GF-K-VG

Ingredients:

- 22oz tomatoes
- 5 tbsp olive oil
- 1/2 cup vegetable stock
- 1/2 tbsp black pepper
- 3 garlic, peeled and chopped
- 3-4 tbsp almonds flakes, roasted
- 1/2 tsp sea salt
- 4 tbsp greek yogurt

Method

1. Heat a large pan over medium heat.

2. Add the oil, chopped tomatoes and garlic. Sprinkle some salt and pepper and roast for 30 seconds.

3. Pour the vegetable stock and simmer for 10 minutes.

4. Transfer this to a blender and puree well—strain into a container.

5. Just before serving, warm the soup and pour it into individual serving bowls. You can also add a little water if the soup is too thick.

6. Garnish with roasted almond flakes and a tablespoon of greek yogurt.

7. Sprinkle some salt and pepper to taste.

NUTRITION FACTS

SERVINGS: 4

amount per serving			DV%			DV%
CALORIES **187**	Total Fat	18 g	23%	Total Carbohydrates	7 g	3%
	Saturated Fat	2.7 g	13%	Dietary Fiber	2.1 g	8%
NET CARBS **4.9 g**	Cholesterol	0 mg	0%	Total Sugars	4.5 g	
	Sodium	251 mg	11%	Protein	2.3 g	

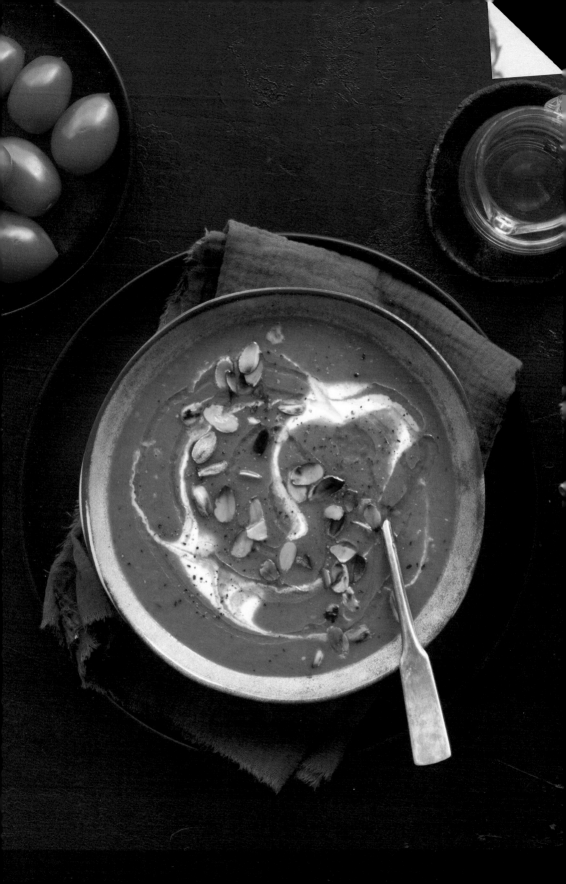

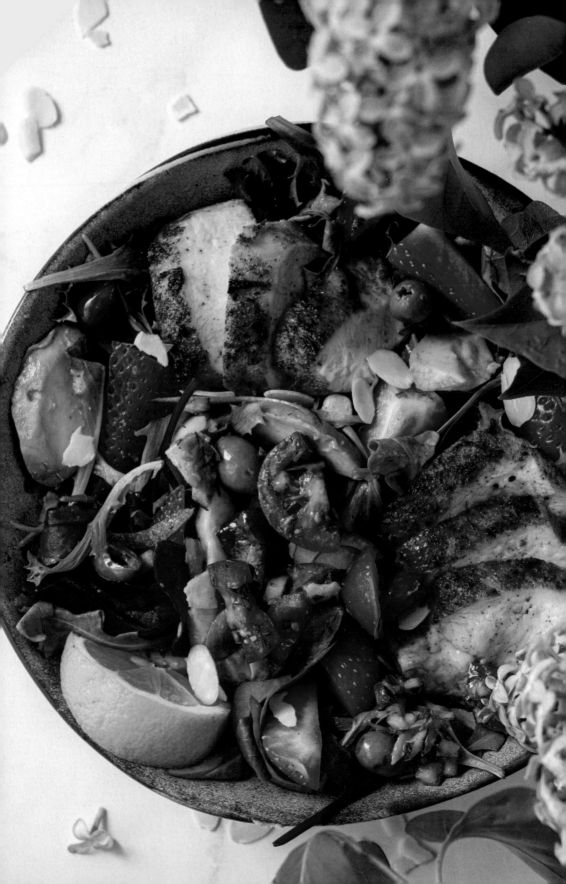

Chicken Salad with Avocado Salsa

Prep Time: 10 minutes | *Cook Time: 40 minutes* | *Total Time: 50 minutes*

4 Servings

GF-K

Ingredients:

- 2 skinless chicken breasts
- 6 cups mixed salad greens
- 8 big strawberries, quartered
- 1 avocado, chunks
- 3-4 thinly sliced red onion rings
- 3 tbsp olives
- 2 tbsp almonds flakes

- 2 tbsp parsley, chopped
- 1 lemon, quartered
- 4 tbsp extra virgin olive oil
- 1 tbsp paprika powder
- 2 tsp salt
- 1/2 tsp black pepper

Method

1. Whisk the extra virgin olive oil, kosher salt, paprika, and freshly ground black pepper in a small bowl until combined.

2. Place the chicken breasts in a shallow bowl with half of the olive oil mixture, cover and refrigerate for 30 minutes.

3. Add some oil to a grill or non-stick pan and set heat to medium-high. Cook chicken for 3 minutes, then flip and cook for another 3 minutes. The chicken is finished when it hits 165 degrees internal temperature. Let the chicken rest for 5 minutes, then slice into 1/4 inch slices.

4. Arrange the spinach, olives, strawberries and red onion in a bowl and toss with the rest of the olive oil mixture. Add the avocado, sliced chicken and top with almond slices and quartered lemon. Serve immediately.

NUTRITION FACTS

SERVINGS: 4

amount per serving			DV%			DV%
CALORIES **550**	Total Fat	45.6 g	58%	Total Carbohydrates	15.8 g	6%
	Saturated Fat	7.8 g	39%	Dietary Fiber	6.4 g	23%
NET CARBS **9.4 g**	Cholesterol	65 mg	39%	Total Sugars	5.6 g	
	Sodium	124 mg	5%	Protein	23.9 g	

Cauliflower Pizza

Prep Time: 15 minutes | *Cook Time: 35 minutes* | *Total Time: 50 minutes*

1 Serving
GF

Ingredients:

- 1.5 pounds cauliflower, florets
- 1/2 cup shredded cheddar cheese
- 1 egg, beaten
- 1 teaspoon oregano

- salt and pepper to taste
- 1 cup shredded mozzarella
- 1 1/2 cup tomato sauce
- spicy salami

Method

1. Preheat your oven to 400°F.
2. Remove the cauliflower florets from the stem and grate them by hand or using a food processor.
3. Sauté the grated cauliflower in a pan on medium heat for around 10 minutes and let it cool.
4. Transfer the cauliflower into a thin kitchen towel and squeeze it as hard as you can until all the excess moisture is out.
5. Into a mixing bowl, add the drained cauliflower, cheese, egg and seasonings. Use your hands to combine everything, forming a pizza dough.
6. Line a baking sheet with parchment paper (or use a pizza stone) and form the dough into an even circle.
7. Bake for 25 minutes, or until lightly golden, remove from oven, add the toppings and bake for an additional 10 minutes.

NUTRITION FACTS

SERVINGS: 1

amount per serving			DV%			DV%
CALORIES **506**	Total Fat	19.2 g	25%	Total Carbohydrates	57.7 g	21%
	Saturated Fat	4.6 g	23%	Dietary Fiber	22.5 g	80%
NET CARBS **35.2 g**	Cholesterol	179 mg	60%	Total Sugars	32.3 g	
	Sodium	2361 mg	103%	Protein	38.9 g	

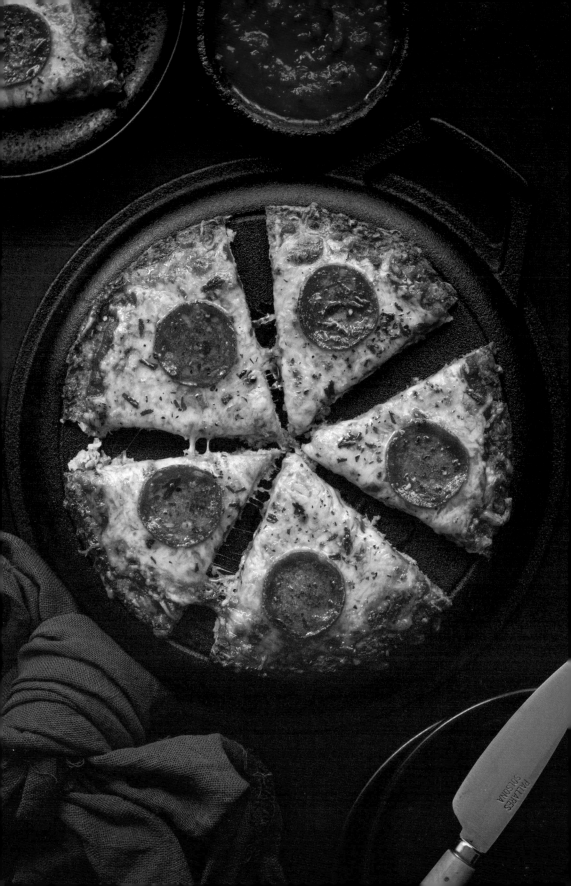

APPETIZERS

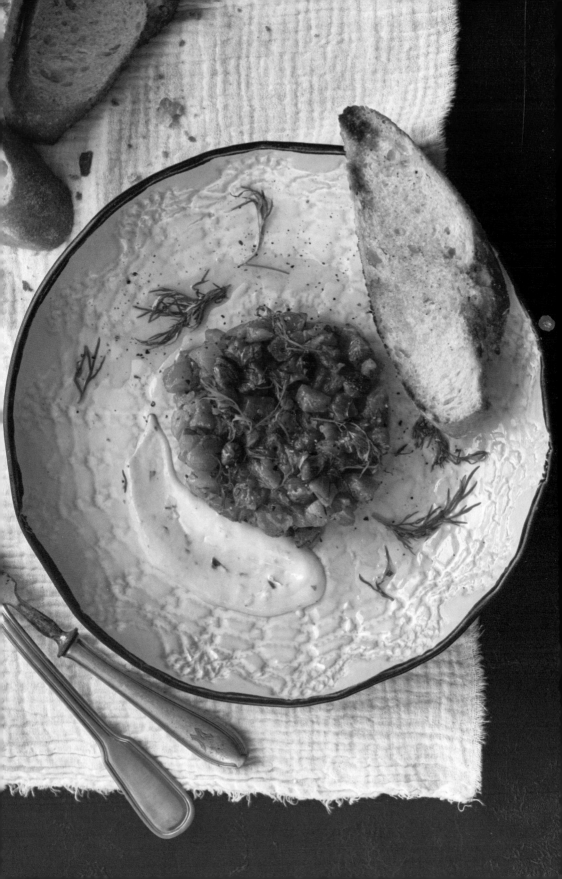

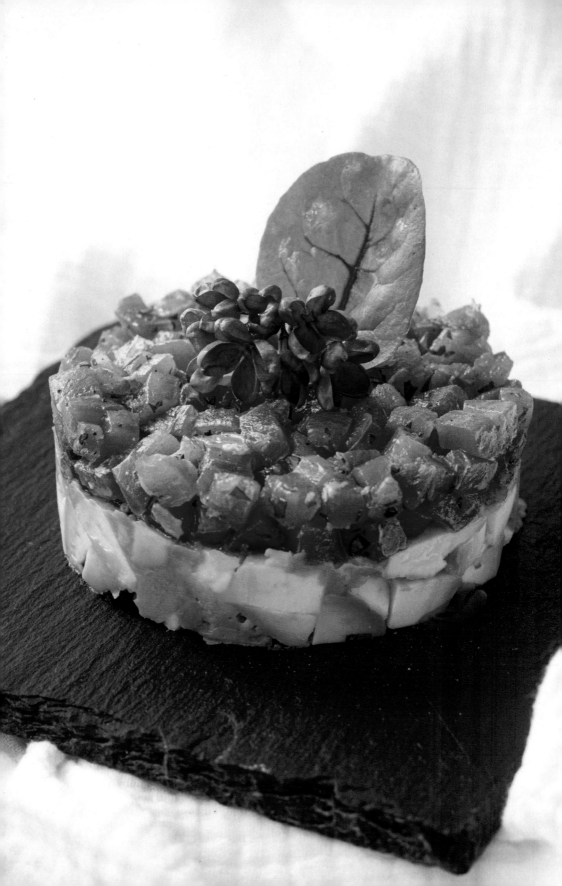

Keto Tuna Tartare

Prep Time: 20 minutes | Total Time: 30 minutes

4 Servings

GF-K

Ingredients

- 1 pound fresh tuna
- 2 avocados
- 1 tbsp parsley, chopped
- 2 tsp ginger, grated

- 1 lime, zest + juice
- 1 tbsp soy sauce
- 4 tbsp Extra Virgin Olive Oil
- Salt & pepper

Method

1. Place tuna in the freezer for 15 minutes before step 2.
2. Cut the tuna into even cubes, as big or small as you prefer.
3. In a small mixing bowl, stir together soy sauce, lime juice, lime zest, ginger, parsley, olive oil and salt & pepper.
4. Add the tuna cubes to the sauce and stir until evenly coated. Cover and refrigerate.
5. Chop the avocado into 1/2" pieces.
6. Start assembling the tower by pressing the avocado into the bottom of a ring mould.
7. Add the tuna mix on top of the avocado and slowly remove the mould.
8. Serve with The No Sugar Company Keto Bread.

NUTRITION FACTS

SERVINGS: 4

amount per serving			DV%			DV%
CALORIES **442**	Total Fat	34.9 g	45%	Total Carbohydrates	8.9 g	3%
	Saturated Fat	6.1 g	31%	Dietary Fiber	6.8 g	24%
NET CARBS **2.1 g**	Cholesterol	48 mg	16%	Total Sugars	0.6 g	
	Sodium	270 mg	12%	Protein	27.2 g	

Keto Baked Brie with Berries & Nuts

Prep Time: 15 minutes | *Cook Time: 15 minutes* | *Total Time: 30 minutes*

4 Servings

GF-K-VG

Ingredients

- 1 cup walnuts
- 1 tbsp unsalted butter, melted
- 1 brie wheel, 13.2 oz

- 3 tbsp balsamic glaze (optional)
- 1/3 cup raspberries
- No Sugar Company Keto Bread for dipping

Method

1. Preheat oven to 350°F and line a baking sheet with parchment paper and set nearby.

2. Add walnuts and melted butter to a small saucepan over medium heat, toss the walnuts to coat and cook for 5 minutes until lightly browned, frequently stirring, so it doesn't burn.

3. Set aside and let cool.

4. Place the brie wheel in a rimmed baking dish (or cast-iron skillet). If you don't like the rind, trim off the top layer of the brie.

5. Bake brie for 12-14 minutes or until heated. Remove from oven and allow the brie to cool for 5 minutes.

6. To serve, arrange the raspberries and sprinkle toasted walnuts on top of the baked brie.

7. Optional: drizzle balsamic glaze generously on and around the brie. Use No Sugar Company Keto Bread for dipping.

NUTRITION FACTS

SERVINGS: 1

amount per serving			DV%			DV%
CALORIES **338**	Total Fat	30.3 g	39%	Total Carbohydrates	6 g	3%
	Saturated Fat	8.4 g	42%	Dietary Fiber	2.8 g	10%
NET CARBS **3.2 g**	Cholesterol	40 mg	13%	Total Sugars	2.4 g	
	Sodium	222 mg	10%	Protein	14.3 g	

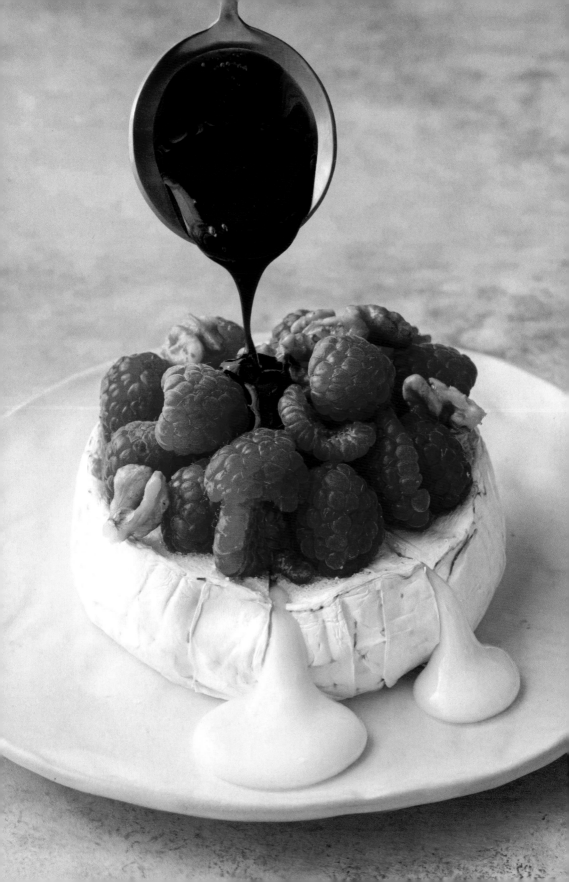

Smoked Salmon Rolls

Prep Time: 15 minutes | *Cook Time: 10 minutes* | *Total Time: 25 minutes*

12 Pieces

GF-K

Ingredients

- 1/2 cup cream cheese
- 2 tbsp chives, minced
- 1 tbsp lemon zest
- 3 tbsp black sesame seeds
- 8 ounces smoked salmon
- 1 medium cucumber
- 1 tsp salt
- 1/2 tsp pepper

Method

1. In a bowl, combine the cream cheese with chives and lemon zest, mix well to get a fluffy consistency—season with salt and pepper.
2. Sprinkle a piece of plastic wrap with the sesame seeds.
3. Place the salmon slices over the sesame seeds, overlap them to form a 10 x 6" rectangle.
4. Spread the whipped cream cheese over the smoked salmon.
5. Place the sliced cucumber along the center of the salmon, use the plastic wrap to help you roll it up.
6. Put into the freezer for 5 minutes for easier cutting.
7. Slice into 12 pieces and serve.

NUTRITION FACTS

SERVINGS: 1

amount per serving			DV%			DV%
CALORIES **41**	Total Fat	3.4 g	4%	Total Carbohydrates	1.8 g	1%
	Saturated Fat	2.1 g	11%	Dietary Fiber	0.3 g	1%
NET CARBS **1.5 g**	Cholesterol	11 mg	4%	Total Sugars	0.8 g	
	Sodium	29 mg	1%	Protein	1.1 g	

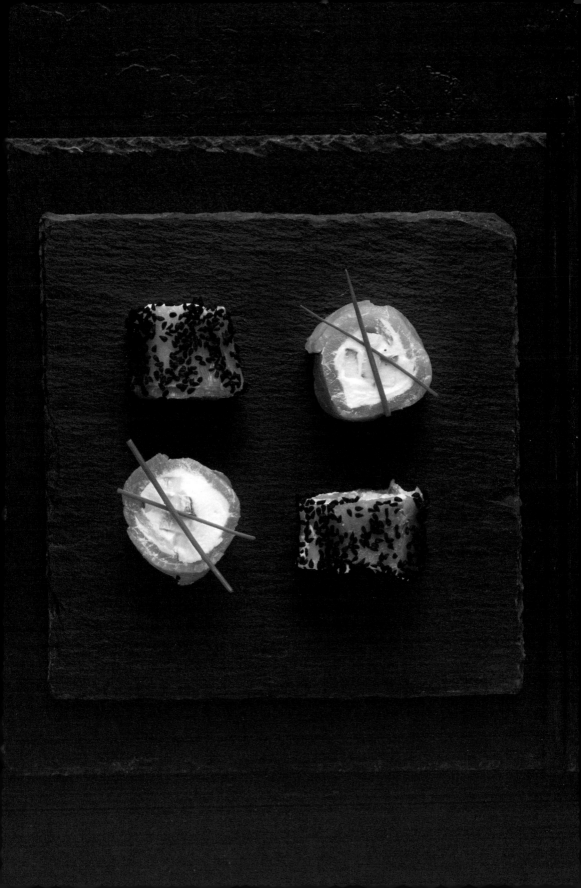

Guacamole with Bacon Chips

Prep Time: 10 minutes | Cook Time: 5 minutes | Total Time: 15 minutes

4 Servings

GF-K

Ingredients

- 2 large avocados, halved and pitted
- 2 tsp lime juice
- 1/2 tsp sea salt
- 1/4 cup red onion, finely chopped
- 2 tbsp parsley, finely chopped
- 5 cherry tomatoes, finely chopped
- 4 slices bacon, diced

Method

1. Dice bacon and cook on medium heat in a skillet until crispy. Set aside.
2. Add avocados, lime, and salt to a large bowl. Mash with a potato masher until smooth with some chunks remaining.
3. Add in red onion, cherry tomatoes, and cilantro. Stir until well mixed.
4. Sprinkle bacon on top of guacamole and serve immediately.

NUTRITION FACTS   SERVINGS: 1

amount per serving			DV%			DV%
CALORIES **338**	Total Fat	27.9 g	36%	Total Carbohydrates	15.6 g	6%
	Saturated Fat	6.8 g	34%	Dietary Fiber	8.7 g	31%
NET CARBS **6.9 g**	Cholesterol	21 mg	7%	Total Sugars	4.8 g	
	Sodium	687 mg	30%	Protein	10.4v g	

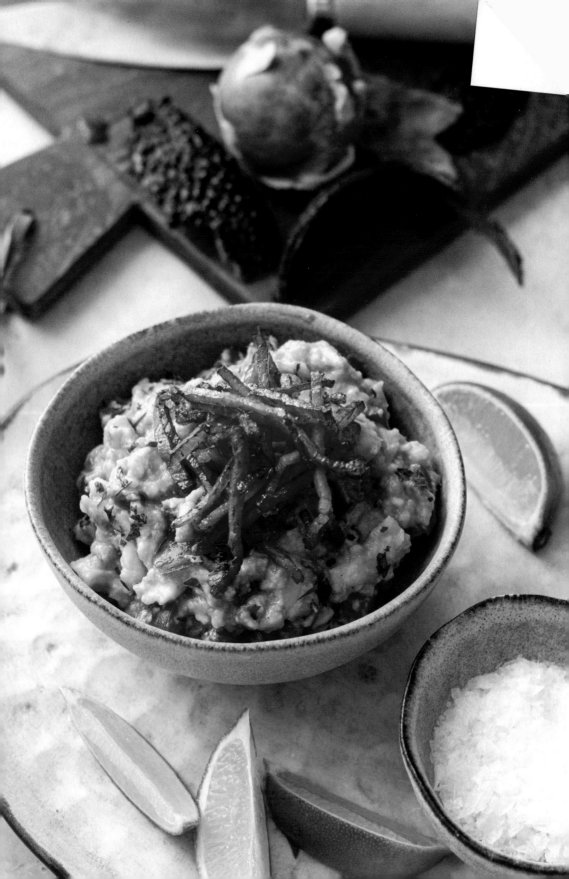

DINNER

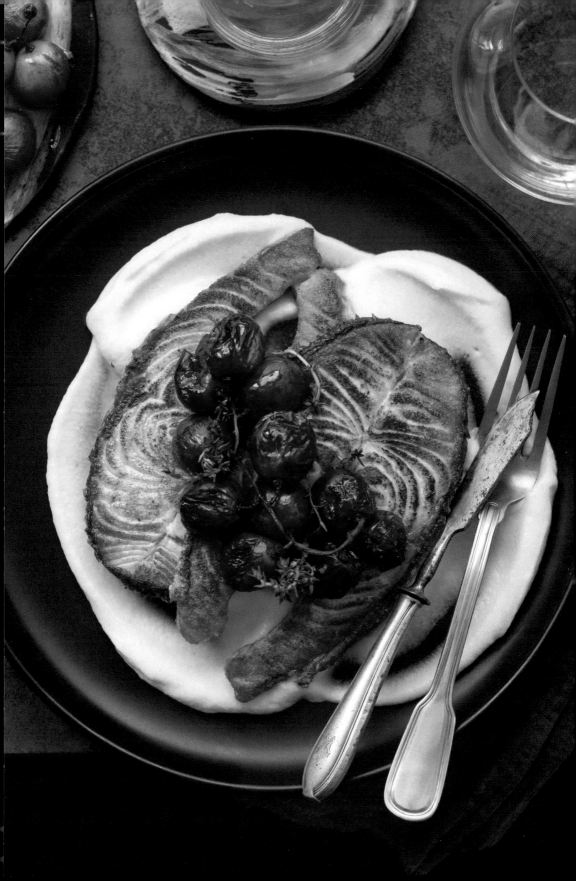

Basil Pesto Pasta

Prep Time: 15 minutes | Cook Time: 5 minutes | Total Time: 20 minutes

6 Servings

VG

Ingredients

- Kosher salt
- 14 ounces (400 grams) dried fusilli pasta
- 1 garlic clove
- 8 ¾ ounces (250 grams) extra-virgin olive oil, plus more
- 3 cups (60g) lightly packed basil leaves

- 1 thyme branch
- 2 ½ ounces (75 grams) finely grated Parmigiano-Reggiano
- 3 ½ ounces (100 grams) freshly ground bread crumbs
- Ice cold water
- Feta and pine-nuts for garnish (optional)

Method

Cook the Pasta

Bring a large pot of water to a boil and season with salt. Add the fusilli to the water and cook, stirring occasionally, until al dente, about eight minutes.

Make the pesto.

While pasta is cooking, make the pesto sauce: Peel garlic and add it to your blender. Pour in olive oil, then add the basil. Strip mint leaves from the stem, and add leaves to blender. Remove as many thyme leaves as you can from the branch, add them to blender. Add half the Parmigiano and half the bread crumbs to the blender. With the blender on, slowly stream in ½ cup of ice-cold water, adding more water by the tablespoonful, until the sauce blends smoothly. Add remaining Parmigiano, season with salt, and blend again until smooth.

When pasta is ready, drain it, reserving at least ½ cup of the cooking water but discarding the herb stems. Return the drained pasta to the pot, and stir in pesto sauce along with more olive oil (about 1 ounce, or 30 grams) to emulsify the pasta and make it shiny, adding some cooking water by the spoonful to make a creamy, silky sauce.

Garnish with some feta and pine-nuts (optional)

NUTRITION FACTS

SERVINGS: 6

amount per serving			DV%			DV%
CALORIES **677**	Total Fat	43.3 g	56%	Total Carbohydrates	62.1 g	23%
	Saturated Fat	7.7 g	39%	Dietary Fiber	3.3 g	12%
NET CARBS **58.8 g**	Cholesterol	9 mg	3%	Total Sugars	2.6 g	
	Sodium	238 mg	10%	Protein	15.2 g	

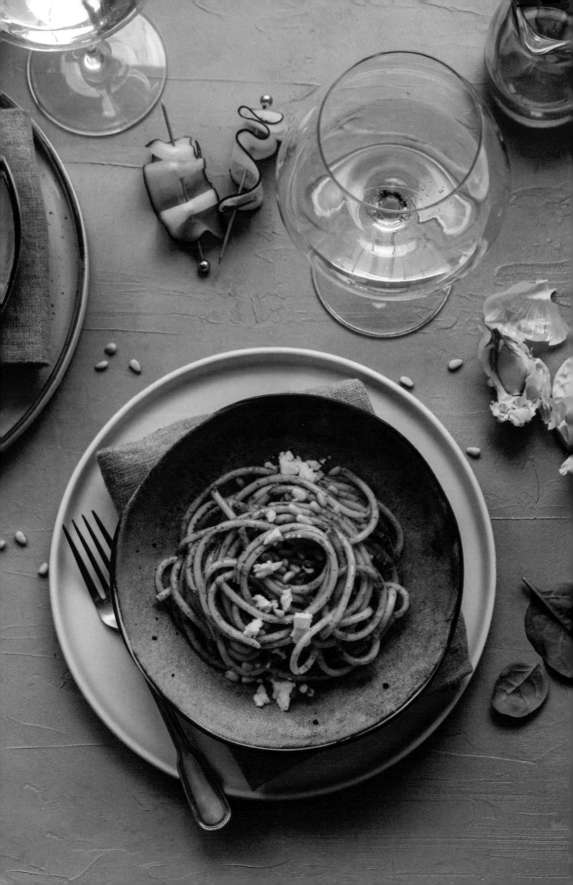

Salmon Steak

Prep Time: 15 minutes | *Cook Time: 35 minutes* | *Total Time: 50 minutes*

8 Servings

GF-K

Ingredients

Ingredients for grapes and salmon.

- 1 large bunch red seedless grapes
- 2 tablespoons olive oil divided
- 4 sprigs thyme plus more for garnish
- Salt and pepper to taste
- 1 pound Wild Atlantic Salmon

Ingredients for cauliflower puree

- 17 oz cauliflower (about 1 medium head)
- ¼ cup water
- 6 tbsp unsalted butter
- 6 tbsp your choice of milk
- 1 tsp salt

METHOD

1. Preheat oven to 375°F. Place grapes on a baking tray and toss with 1 tablespoon of olive oil. Season lightly with salt and pepper. Roast grapes for around 15-20 minutes or until the grapes start to burst, have slightly blistered skin and have shrunk in size. Remove from heat and set aside.
2. In the meantime make your puree. Roughly chop cauliflower into thin slices that are about a tenth of an inch thick.
3. Place cauliflower, water, butter, and salt in a saucepan and cover with lid.
4. Begin heating on high then reduce heat to medium and continue steaming until cauliflower is tender and there is little water left in the pot.
5. Add cauliflower, milk and butter to a blender and blend until very smooth. Season to taste and set aside covered with lid.
6. Season salmon with salt and pepper, add remaining oil to a cast iron skillet over medium high heat. When oil is hot, add salmon and cook for about 2-3 minutes on each side.
7. Spoon puree over your plate, add salmon and top with roasted grapes.
   Garnish with fresh thyme leaves. Enjoy!

NUTRITION FACTS

SERVINGS: 6

amount per serving			DV%			DV%
CALORIES **457**	Total Fat	35 g	45%	Total Carbohydrates	13.1 g	5%
	Saturated Fat	14.2 g	71%	Dietary Fiber	3.8 g	14%
NET CARBS **9.3 g**	Cholesterol	128 mg	43%	Total Sugars	8.6 g	
	Sodium	1298 mg	56%	Protein	27.9 g	

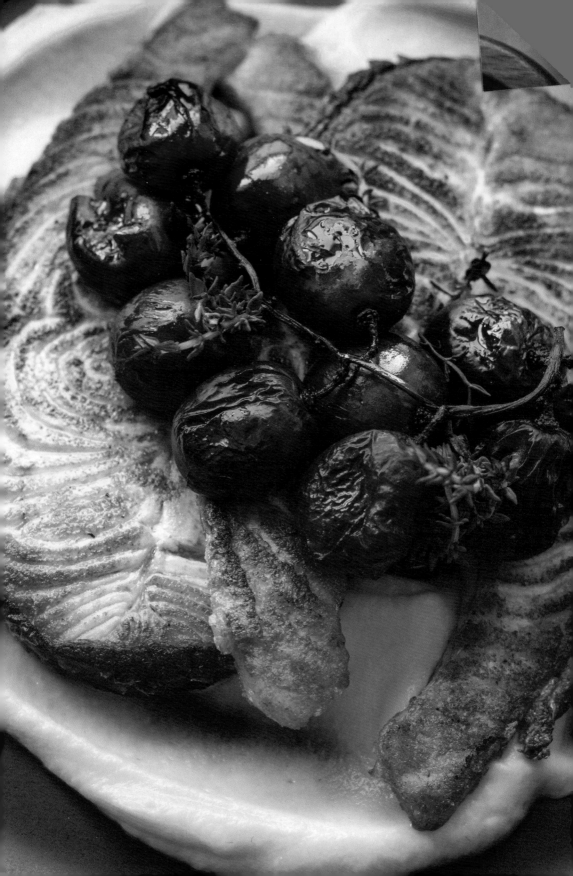

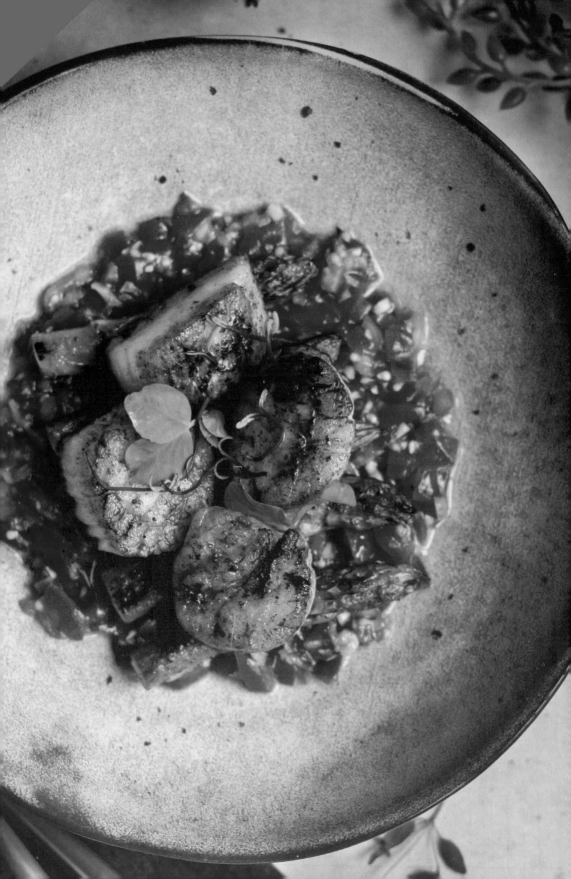

Summer Scallops

Prep Time: 15 minutes | Cook Time: 15 minutes | Total Time: 30 minutes

4 Servings

GF-K

Ingredients

- 16 large Scallops
- 20 green Asparagus
- 20 oz Cherry Tomatoes finely diced
- Garlic, minced

- Basil
- Salt and Pepper
- Olive Oil

METHOD

1. Mix tomatoes, garlic, basil and season with salt, pepper and olive oil to taste.

2. Tail the asparagus and char them in a hot pan for about 2 minutes.

3. Heat an oiled skillet or pan until it's sizzling.

4. The first scallop should sizzle as soon as it hits the oil. If it doesn't, wait and let pan continue heating before adding any more.

5. Use a large pan to avoid over crowding, or cook in batches to make sure they are at least 1-inch apart.

6. Sear them without moving them for about 2-3 minutes on each side. You will want the scallops to sizzle and crisp to a golden color on the outside. Done!

7. Complete the dish by assembling all of the ingredients as shown in the picture and can serve with cauliflower mash (included in our Salmon Steak recipe).

NUTRITION FACTS

SERVINGS: 6

amount per serving			DV%			DV%
CALORIES **460**	Total Fat	20.2 g	26%	Total Carbohydrates	43.8 g	16%
	Saturated Fat	2.9 g	14%	Dietary Fiber	19.1 g	68%
NET CARBS **24.7 g**	Cholesterol	40 mg	13%	Total Sugars	12.6 g	
	Sodium	237 mg	10%	Protein	39.9 g	

Roasted Chicken

Prep Time: 20 minutes | Cook Time: 60 minutes | Total Time: 90 minutes

2 Servings
GF-K

Ingredients

- 3-pound whole chicken, cleaned
- ½ white onion, peeled and halved lengthwise
- ½ lemon, halved lengthwise
- ½ fennel bulb, halved lengthwise
- 4 sprigs Thai basil
- 2 egg yolks
- 3 tablespoons crushed black pepper
- 3 tablespoons smoked paprika
- 4 tablespoons of lemon salt

Method
Preheat oven to 400°F. Allow chicken to come to room temperature before preparing. Stand chicken neck side down on a sheet tray with legs upwards and facing you. Season cavity of the chicken with 1 to 2 tablespoons of lemon salt. Stuff the onion, lemon, and fennel wedges into the cavity so that it will hold its shape and not collapse while roasting. Stuff Thai basil bunch last, into center of the cavity with the leaves facing outward.

Whisk the egg yolks together to make an egg wash. Brush the chicken liberally with the egg wash over any visible part of chicken skin, minus backside of the chicken. This will act as a glue for the seasoning to stick.

Sprinkle 3 tablespoons of pepper and paprika and 4 tablespoons lemon salt over every inch of the chicken. Be sure to spread open the wings and legs and rub seasoning in all the crevasses to ensure maximum flavor in the meat and drippings.

Trussing
Cut approximately a 2-foot piece of butchers' twine.

Wrap the twine around chicken lengthwise so the middle section of the twine is at neck area and each side of the twine is touching the wings and the thighs (under the drumstick). Bring the twine ends together and cross and then wrap the other way.

Tighten the twine and finish by tying the ends together into a bow. Make sure twine is holding the wings and legs in place tight enough to ensure a plump shape for the chicken during roasting.

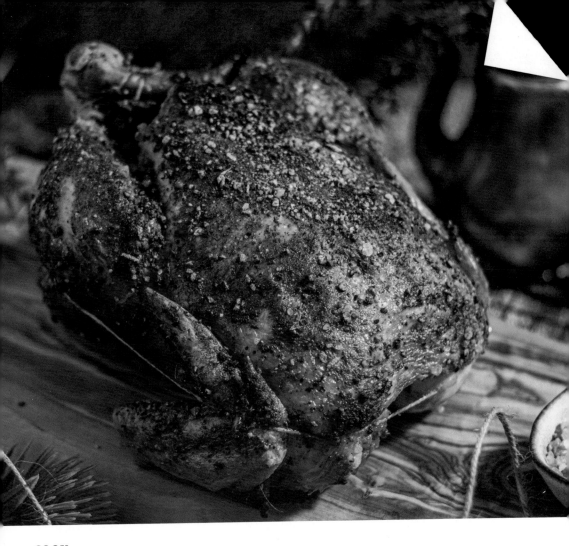

COOK

Place a wire rack between chicken and the sheet tray to ensure that even the bottom of the chicken skin gets crisp. Roast in the center rack of the oven for 60 minutes, or until the internal temperature of the chicken breast area reaches 165°F. Remove from oven and rest for 10 minutes.

This is great to serve with roasted vegetables. Should you have any leftovers, they can be leveraged in lettuce wraps or chicken soup.

NUTRITION FACTS

SERVINGS: 2

amount per serving			DV%			DV%
CALORIES **673**	Total Fat	27.5 g	35%	Total Carbohydrates	0.3 g	0%
	Saturated Fat	7.8 g	39%	Dietary Fiber	0 g	0%
NET CARBS **0.3 g**	Cholesterol	408 mg	136%	Total Sugars	0.1 g	
	Sodium	297 mg	13%	Protein	99.8 g	

Mussels Fra Diavolo

Prep Time: 30 minutes | Cook Time: 15 minutes | Total Time: 45 minutes

4 Servings

GF-K

Ingredients

- 2 tbsp extra virgin olive oil
- 1 large shallot, minced
- 2 cloves garlic, thinly sliced
- 1 tsp crushed red pepper flakes (omit if you don't like spicy)
- 1 cup white wine
- 1 can San Marzano canned Tomatoes (14 oz., Polpa)
- 2 lbs fresh mussels, scrubbed clean, with beards removed
- Chopped fresh parsley
- Lemon

Method

1. Heat the olive oil in a large pot over medium-high heat.
2. Add shallots, garlic and red pepper and cook for about 5 minutes or until the shallots are golden, stirring frequently.
3. Stir in white wine and cook until reduced by half.
4. Stir in canned tomatoes, reduce heat to medium-low and simmer for about 5 minutes.
5. Add mussels to pot and stir gently to distribute them evenly within the sauce.
6. Cover and cook for 5 minutes. Gently shake the pan a couple of times during cooking, without removing the cover, to redistribute mussels.
7. After 5 minutes, remove cover from the pan to check mussels. Most should be open. If some remain closed, cover and cook for an additional 2 minutes. At this time, if any mussels are still closed, discard them.
8. Arrange the mussels in a shallow serving bowl and pour sauce over them.
9. Serve your delicious Mussels with crusty bread, lemon wedges and garnish with fresh parsley.

NUTRITION FACTS

SERVINGS: 4

amount per serving			DV%			DV%
CALORIES **312**	Total Fat	12.2 g	16%	Total Carbohydrates	11.8 g	4%
	Saturated Fat	2 g	10%	Dietary Fiber	0.5 g	2%
NET CARBS **11.3 g**	Cholesterol	64 mg	21%	Total Sugars	0.5 g	
	Sodium	685 mg	30%	Protein	27.4 g	

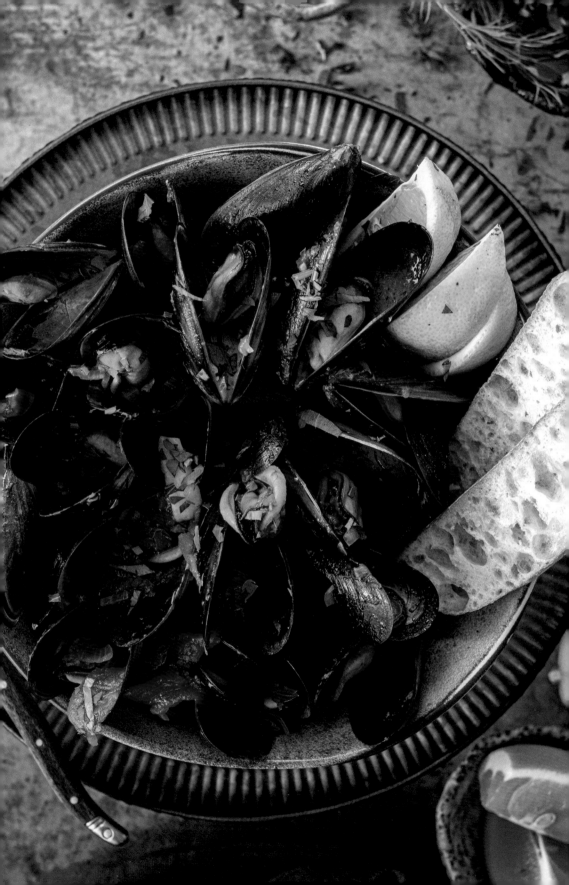

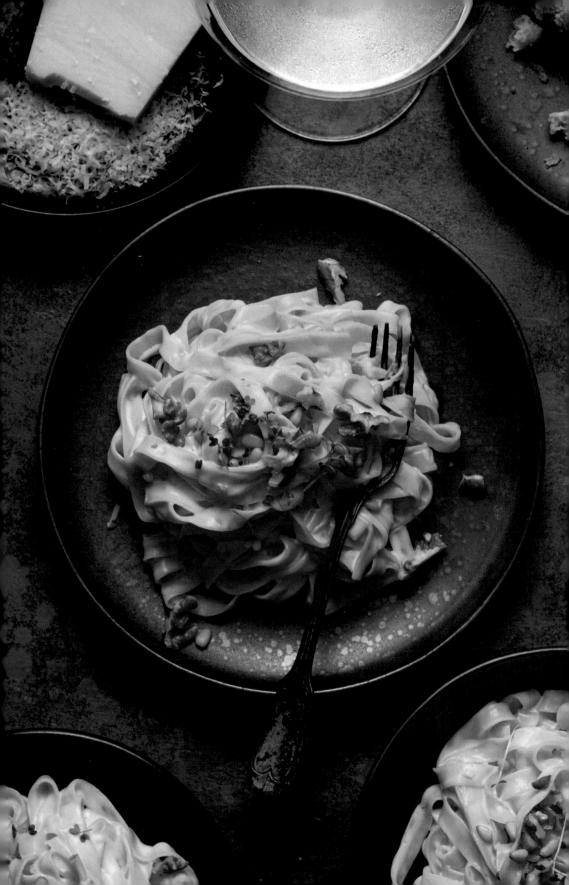

Keto Alfredo Pasta

Prep Time: 5 minutes | Cook Time: 10 minutes | Total Time: 15 minutes

4 Servings

GF-K

Ingredients:

- 2 tbsp butter
- 1 tsp crushed garlic
- 1/4 tsp. Salt
- 1/8 tsp. Pepper
- 3 oz Cream Cheese

- 1 cup Heavy Cream
- 1/2 cup Parmesan
- 2 tablespoons chopped walnuts
- Low Carb Tagliatelle
- Sprouts for garnish

Method

1. In a nonstick pan, melt the butter over medium heat with the garlic.
2. Add in the cream cheese, stirring until melted, then add in the remaining ingredients, stirring until smooth.
3. Simmer for 5-10 minutes, constantly stirring until the sauce has thickened.
4. Combine with low-carb tagliatelle and garnish with chopped walnuts and sprouts.

NUTRITION FACTS

SERVINGS: 4

amount per serving			DV%			DV%
CALORIES **340**	Total Fat	31.6 g	40%	Total Carbohydrates	2.3 g	1%
	Saturated Fat	19.9 g	99%	Dietary Fiber	0 g	0%
NET CARBS **2.3 g**	Cholesterol	99 mg	33%	Total Sugars	0.3 g	
	Sodium	99 mg	25%	Protein	12.4 g	

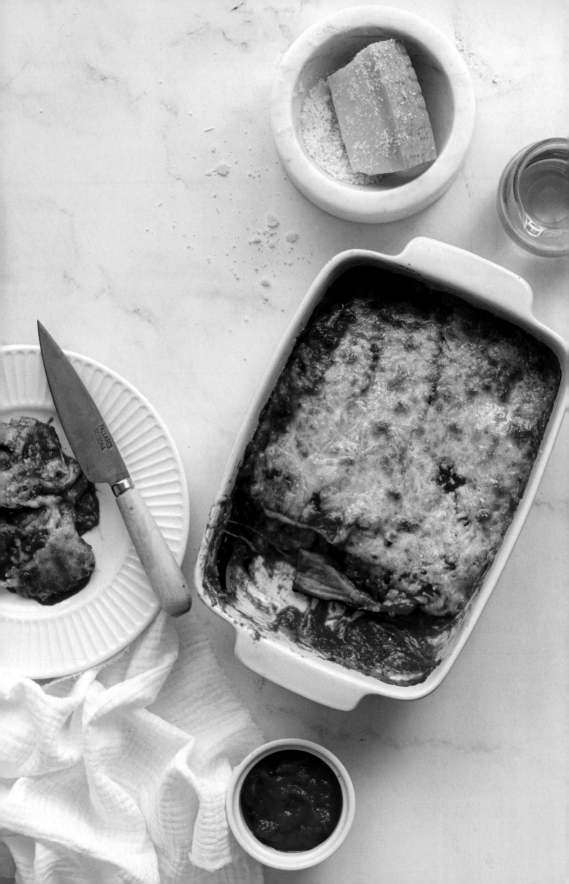

Keto Lasagna

Prep Time: 15 minutes | Cook Time: 55 minutes | Total Time: 1h 10 minutes

4 Servings
GF-K-VG

Ingredients:

- 3 eggplants, approximately 1 1/2 pounds
- 2 tsp salt
- 3 tbsp extra-virgin olive oil
- 1 tsp oregano

- 2 1/2 cups shredded mozzarella,
- 1/2 cup grated Parmesan cheese,
- 1 1/2 cups tomato sauce, seasoned

Method

1. Slice the eggplants lengthwise into 1/4" thick planks and sprinkle with salt. Let stand for 15 minutes, the salt pulls out the bitterness, and you can wipe away the salty moisture with a paper towel.

2. In the meantime, preheat the oven to 400°F.

3. Place the eggplant on a baking sheet lined with parchment paper and brush it lightly with olive oil. Roast in the oven for 15-20 minutes, until spongy and light brown.

4. On the bottom of a 9x13" baking dish, spread around 1/4 cup of the tomato sauce, arrange approximately 6 slices of eggplant on the sauce.

5. Combine mozzarella and parmesan and sprinkle 1/3 of the cheese mix.

6. Repeat this 2-3 times or until you run out of ingredients. Make sure that the last two layers are tomato sauce topped with cheese and oregano.

7. Cover the baking dish tightly with aluminum foil and bake for 20 minutes. Remove the foil and continue for another 20 minutes or until the cheese is golden brown.

8. Let rest for 15-20 minutes before serving. You can freeze the whole dish perfectly once it is cooled down.

NUTRITION FACTS

SERVINGS: 4

amount per serving			DV%			DV%
CALORIES **329**	Total Fat	18.4 g	24%	Total Carbohydrates	33.2 g	12%
	Saturated Fat	5.1 g	26%	Dietary Fiber	14.6 g	52%
NET CARBS **18.6 g**	Cholesterol	16 mg	5%	Total Sugars	17.9 g	
	Sodium	1157 mg	50%	Protein	12.5 g	

Crispy Pork Belly

Prep Time: 10 minutes | Cook Time: 2 hours | Total Time: 2h 10 minutes

8 Servings
GF-K

Ingredients For the crust:

- 2 pounds pork belly, skin-on
- 3 tbsp kosher salt
- 2 tsp freshly ground black pepper
- Some rosemary, minced
- Some thyme, minced
- 1 tsp chilli flakes

Ingredients For the FILLING:

- 5 large eggs
- 1/3 cup lemon juice
- 1/2 cup erythritol
- 2 tbsp coconut flour
- 1/4 cup unsalted butter, melted

Method

1. Use a skin-on pork belly. It gives the crunchy skin we all love!

2. Pat the skin dry with a paper towel and use a sharp knife to score in a diamond-shaped pattern.

3. Be careful to only cut through the skin and fat, don't go too deep and hit the meat.

4. Season your pork belly with salt, freshly ground black pepper, rosemary, chilli flakes and thyme.

5. Ideally, you should do this the day before and refrigerate overnight to get the most flavour into the pork. If not, allow at least 2 hours.

6. Preheat your grill to 450°F.

7. Roast the pork belly for 30 minutes, positioned dead centre on your grill, skin side up, then reduce to 275°F and roast for 1 1/2 hour or more, until tender.

8. Cut into desired pieces and crisp each side in a cast-iron skillet or directly on your grill.

9. You can also deep fry them to get all-around crispiness, but be careful because the juicy pork will make the oil splash around. Cover with a lid.

NUTRITION FACTS

SERVINGS: 8

amount per serving			DV%			DV%
CALORIES **400**	Total Fat	25.5 g	37%	Total Carbohydrates	0.3 g	0%
	Saturated Fat	9.5 g	48%	Dietary Fiber	0.1 g	1%
NET CARBS **0.2 g**	Cholesterol	0 mg	0%	Total Sugars	0 g	
	Sodium	2626 mg	114%	Protein	9.1 g	

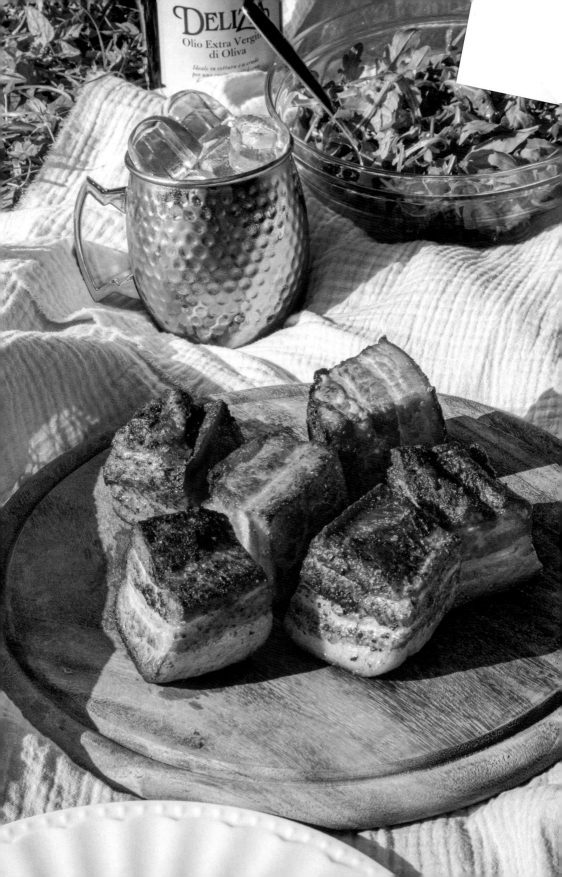

Cordon Bleu

Prep Time: 10 minutes | Cook Time: 30 minutes | Total Time: 40 minutes

4-6 Servings
GF-K

Ingredients:

- 24 oz Chicken breasts
- 1 1/2 cup Pork Panko
- 4 oz Butter
- 6 oz Cream Cheese
- 3 tbsp Mustard

- 6 slices of Swiss cheese
- 1 tbsp olive oil
- salt to taste
- pepper to taste
- garlic powder to taste

Method

1. Preheat the oven to 350°F.
2. Place chicken on parchment paper and season with salt, pepper, and garlic powder.
3. Cut each chicken breast width-wise, almost in half, but not all the way through.
4. Place the second sheet of parchment paper or foil over the halved chicken breast and flatten with a mallet or the bottom of a saucepan.
5. In a saucepan over medium heat, melt the butter, cream cheese, and mustard.
6. Spread the mixture onto the open chicken breasts.
7. Layer cheese slices on top of the mixture.
8. Fold the top of the chicken back down and close with a toothpick or kitchen twine.
9. Place chicken in a large roasting pan and bake for 15-20 minutes.
10. Remove from oven and serve.

NUTRITION FACTS

SERVINGS: 8

amount per serving			DV%			DV%
CALORIES **582**	Total Fat	44 g	56%	Total Carbohydrates	2.7 g	1%
	Saturated Fat	23.6 g	118%	Dietary Fiber	0.3 g	1%
NET CARBS **2.4 g**	Cholesterol	199 mg	66%	Total Sugars	0.5 g	
	Sodium	460 mg	20%	Protein	43 g	

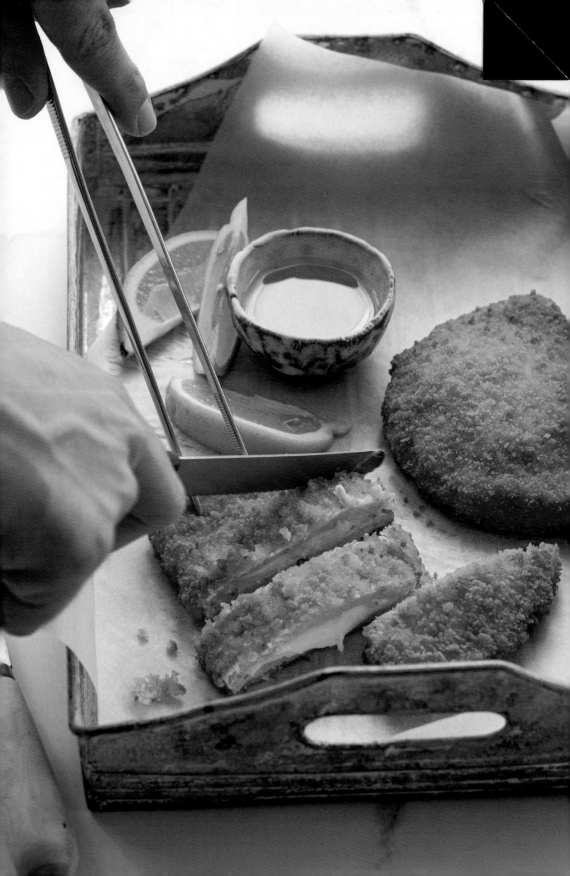

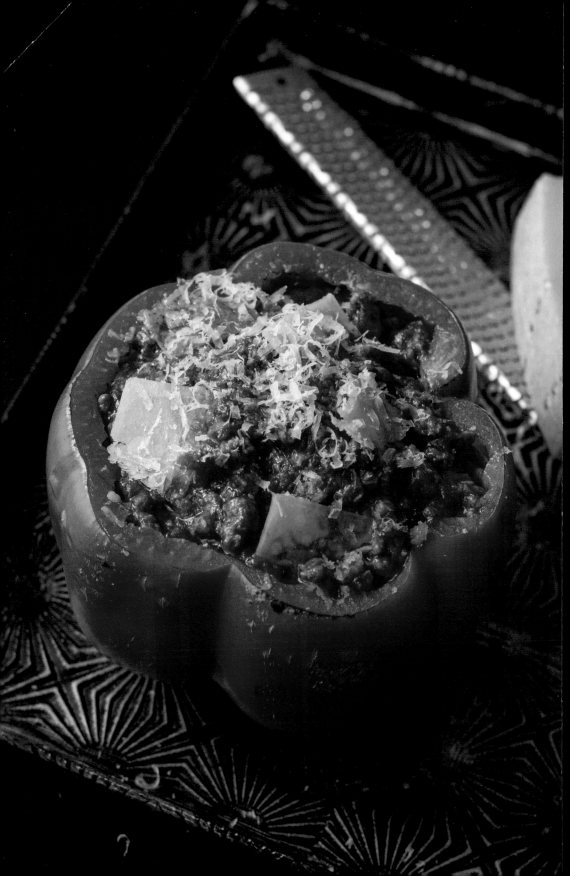

Stuffed Red Bell Peppers

Prep Time: 10 minutes | Cook Time: 25 minutes | Total Time: 35 minutes

4 Servings

GF-K

Ingredients:

- 1 pound ground beef
- 4 bell peppers
- 1/2 cup onion, minced
- 2 teaspoons garlic, minced
- 14 ounces canned tomatoes

- 3 tablespoons tomato paste
- 1 cup parmesan cheese
- 2 teaspoons oregano
- 1 teaspoon salt
- 1/2 teaspoon black pepper

Method

1. Preheat the oven to 475°F.

2. Cut the tops off the bell peppers and use a spoon to remove the membranes and seeds.

3. Arrange peppers in an oiled baking dish and cover them tightly with aluminum foil.

4. Prebake the peppers for 15 minutes.

5. Meanwhile, heat a tbsp of olive oil in a large nonstick pan and add the ground beef, onion, and garlic. Sauté for 2 to 3 minutes, stirring occasionally.

6. Stir in tomatoes, tomato paste, dried oregano, salt, black pepper, and cook for 3 minutes until heated through, stirring occasionally.

7. Divide your beef mixture evenly among all peppers and cover with the tops.

8. Bake for approximately 20 minutes, until bell peppers are tender.

9. Finish with high-quality parmesan cheese and a drizzle of extra virgin olive oil.

NUTRITION FACTS

SERVINGS: 4

amount per serving			DV%			DV%
CALORIES **345**	Total Fat	12.1 g	16%	Total Carbohydrates	16.1 g	6%
	Saturated Fat	5.7 g	29%	Dietary Fiber	3.3 g	12%
NET CARBS **12.8 g**	Cholesterol	116 mg	39%	Total Sugars	9.3 g	
	Sodium	578 mg	25%	Protein	43.6 g	

DESSERTS

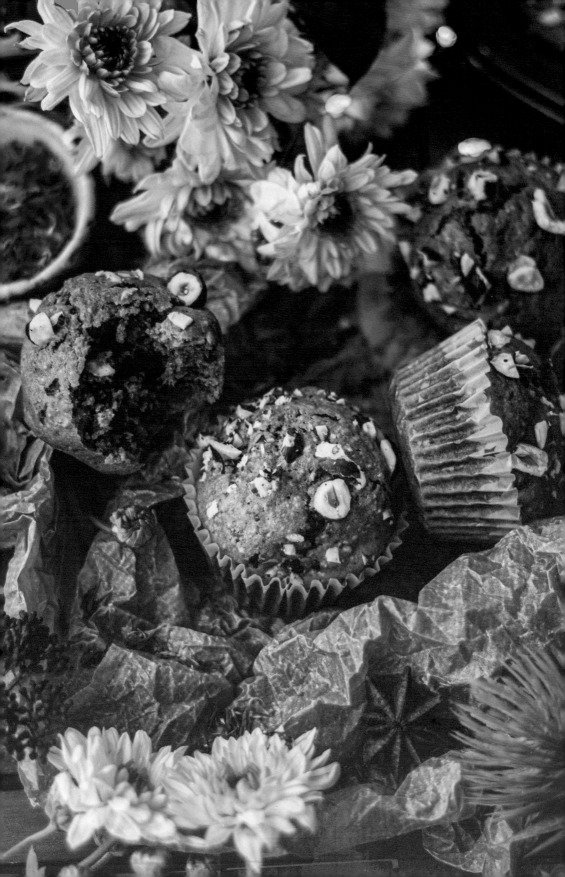

Keto Chocolate Milk

Prep Time: 10 minutes | Cook Time: 0 minutes | Total Time: 10 minutes

2 Servings

GF-K-VG

Ingredients For chocolate milk
- 2 cups of unsweetened milk of choice
- 4 tablespoons cocoa powder
- 4 tablespoons erythritol
- ½ teaspoons vanilla
- Pinch kosher salt

INGREDIENTS FOR WHIPPED CREAM

- 2 cups heavy cream
- 2 teaspoons of erythritol
- 1 tsp vanilla extract

Method

1. For chocolate milk, place all ingredients in a blender and blend until everything has combined.

2. To prepare whipped cream, freeze your mixing bowl for at least 15 minutes.

3. Once chilled, add heavy cream, erythritol, vanilla extract and using a stand mixer, whip together on medium speed, until medium peaks form.

4. Pour your chocolate into 2 glasses, top with generous amount of whipped cream and sprinkle some cocoa powder on top.

NUTRITION FACTS

SERVINGS: 4

amount per serving			DV%			DV%
CALORIES **561**	Total Fat	50.9 g	65%	Total Carbohydrates	21.2 g	8%
	Saturated Fat	31.5 g	158%	Dietary Fiber	3.6 g	3%
NET CARBS **17.6 g**	Cholesterol	184 mg	61%	Total Sugars	11.3 g	
	Sodium	163 mg	7%	Protein	12.6 g	

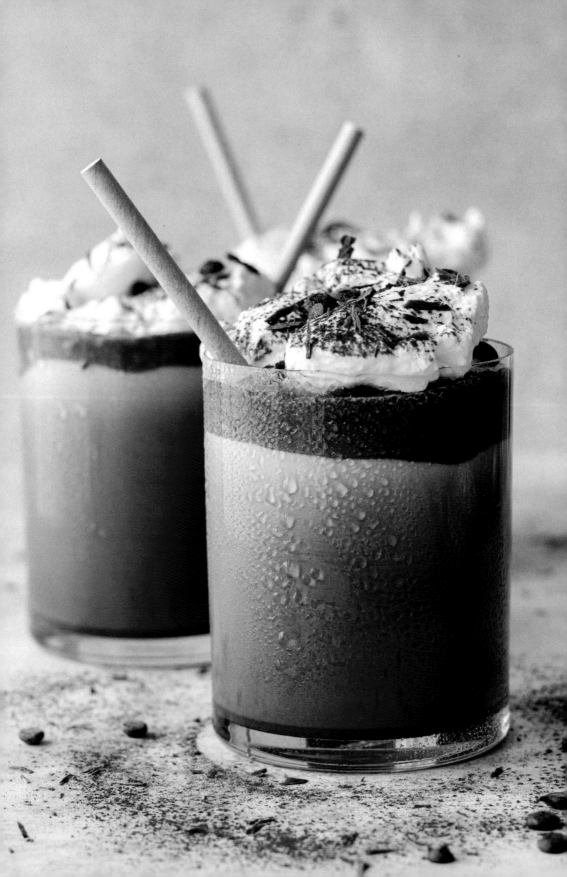

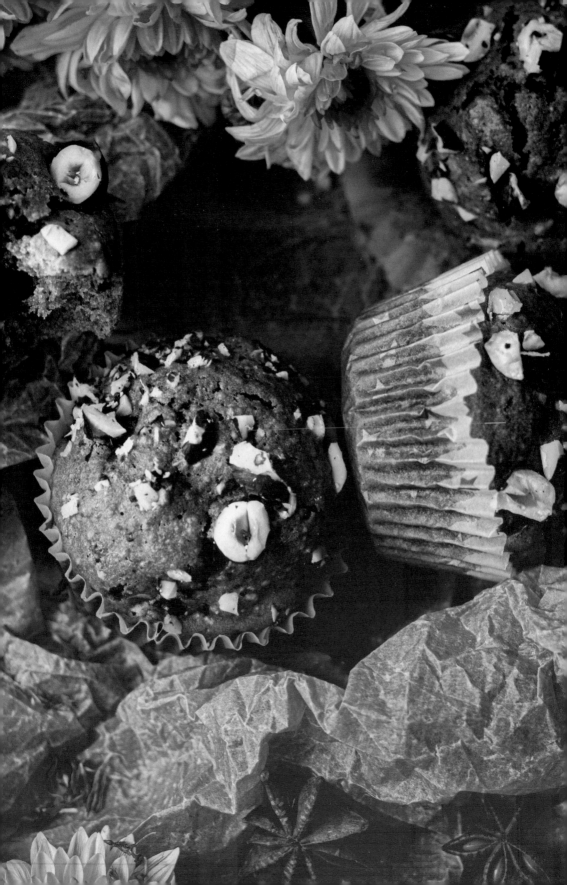

Keto Chocolove Muffins

Prep Time: 5 minutes | Cook Time: 25 minutes | Total Time: 30 minutes

12 Servings
VG

Ingredients

- 1 ¼ cups (190 g) all-purpose flour, divided into three
- 3 Tbsp (15 g) cacao powder
- 2 tsp (10 g) baking powder
- 1 tsp (3 g) cinnamon
- ¼ tsp salt
- 10 g of erythritol
- ¼ tsp ground cardamom

- 1 cup (95 g) almond flour
- ½ cup (50 g) raw walnuts, chopped
- ½ cup (75 g) dried apricots, chopped
- ½ cup (75 g) no sugar chocolate, chopped
- 2 eggs
- ⅓ cup (80 ml) olive oil
- 1 cup (240 ml) of unsweetened milk

Method

1. Preheat oven to 350°F.
2. Combine all the dry ingredients in a large bowl and stir
3. Add all wet ingredients to the same bowl and stir.
4. Divide the batter evenly and bake in the oven for 20 - 25 minutes.

NUTRITION FACTS

SERVINGS: 12

amount per serving			DV%			DV%
CALORIES **225**	Total Fat	16 g	21%	Total Carbohydrates	17.6 g	6%
	Saturated Fat	2.5 g	12%	Dietary Fiber	2.9 g	10%
NET CARBS **14.7 g**	Cholesterol	29 mg	10%	Total Sugars	1.7 g	
	Sodium	21 mg	1%	Protein	7.3 g	

Keto Chia Pudding

Prep Time: 5 minutes | Wait Time: at least 6 hours

4 Servings
GF-K-VG

Ingredients

- 1 ½ cups unsweetened milk
- ½ cup chia seeds
- 1 Tbsp erythritol
- 1 tsp vanilla extract

FOR SERVING

- Fresh fruit
- Whipped cream
- Gingerbread men

Method

1. To a mixing bowl add milk, chia seeds, erythritol and vanilla. Whisk to combine.

2. Cover and refrigerate overnight (or at least 6 hours). The chia pudding should be thick and creamy. If not, add more chia seeds, stir, and refrigerate for another hour or so.

3. Stick thin slices of orange to the side of the glass and pour chia pudding over. Decorate how desired.

NUTRITION FACTS

SERVINGS: 4

amount per serving			DV%			DV%
CALORIES **399**	Total Fat	21.2 g	27%	Total Carbohydrates	39.8 g	14%
	Saturated Fat	4.1 g	21%	Dietary Fiber	19.5 g	70%
NET CARBS **20.3 g**	Cholesterol	15 mg	5%	Total Sugars	14.5 g	
	Sodium	96 mg	4%	Protein	15.4 g	

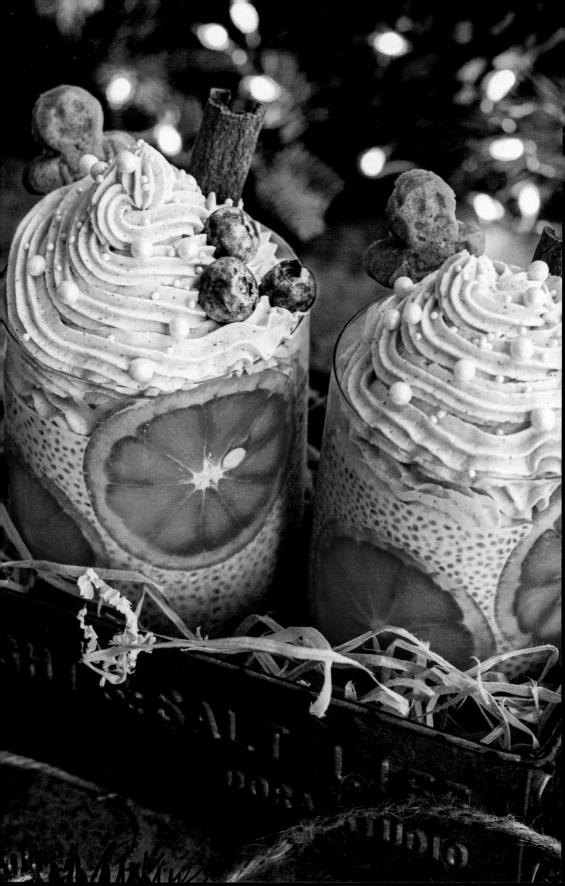

Frosty Chocolate Keto Shake

Prep Time: 10 minutes | Total Time: 10 minutes

2 Servings

GF-K-VG

Ingredients

- 2 tbsp heavy cream
- 1/2 cup almond milk
- 1 medium avocado
- 1/2 tsp vanilla extract
- 4 tbsp cocoa powder
- 1 tbsp chia seeds
- 4-8 tbsp stevia
- 4 No Sugar Keto Cup, Dark Chocolate Caramel
- 1 cup ice cubes
- 2 tbsp almonds, chopped

Method

1. In a small saucepan, melt the keto cups over low heat, add one or two tablespoons of heavy cream if needed. Pour your melted keto cups onto the inside of 2 tall glasses and put them into the fridge to allow the chocolate to firm up.
2. Add almond milk, avocado, vanilla extract, cocoa powder, chia seeds, stevia and ice cubes to a blender. Blend until smooth and thick.
3. Pour into two glasses and top with the almonds and two extra keto cups, chopped.

NUTRITION FACTS

SERVINGS: 4

amount per serving			DV%			DV%
CALORIES **602**	Total Fat	59.4 g	76%	Total Carbohydrates	21.8 g	8%
	Saturated Fat	32 g	160%	Dietary Fiber	13 g	47%
NET CARBS **8.8 g**	Cholesterol	82 mg	27%	Total Sugars	2.8 g	
	Sodium	44 mg	2%	Protein	7.3 g	

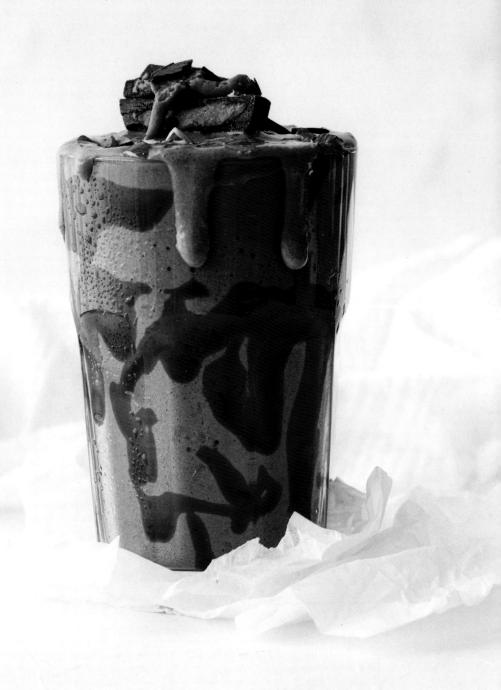

Keto Bomb Brownies

Prep Time: 15 minutes | Cook Time: 20 minutes | Total Time: 35 minutes

12 Servings
GF-K-VG

Ingredients

- 130 g butter
- 170 g powdered erythritol
- 80 g cocoa powder
- 1/2 teaspoon salt
- 2 eggs (room temperature)

- 70 g almond flour
- 12 No Sugar Keto Bombs, peanut butter
- Some flaky sea salt for garnish

  *When baking, always use a kitchen scale and measure in grams

Method

1. Preheat the oven to 350°F.
2. Line the bottom and sides of an 8x8-inch baking pan with parchment paper and set it aside.
3. Add butter, erythritol, cocoa powder and salt to a bowl and melt over a hot water bath, constantly whisking until everything is well incorporated.
4. Remove from heat and allow the mixture to cool slightly.
5. Add one egg at a time, whisking until each one is completely incorporated. The texture should be smooth, and all of the erythritol should dissolve into the mixture.
6. Add the almond flour and whisk until thoroughly combined.
7. Add half of the batter into your baking pan, line with the Keto bombs and cover with the rest of the batter.
8. Bake for 20 minutes, the center with the Keto bombs should be holding their shape with the brownie nicely moist and steaming.
9. Let cool down completely and sprinkle with flakey sea salt (optional).
10. Cut into 12 pieces to have a delicious Keto bomb in the centre of each brownie.

NUTRITION FACTS

SERVINGS: 4

amount per serving			DV%			DV%
CALORIES **196**	Total Fat	18.1 g	14%	Total Carbohydrates	12.3 g	7%
	Saturated Fat	5.7 g	29%	Dietary Fiber	2.4 g	9%
NET CARBS **9.9 g**	Cholesterol	48 mg	16%	Total Sugars	0.2 g	
	Sodium	164 mg	7%	Protein	5 g	

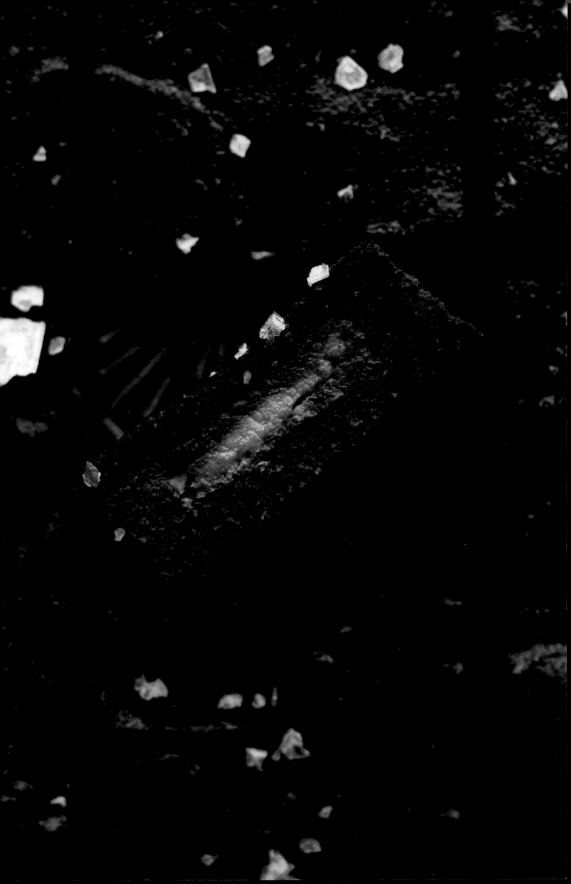

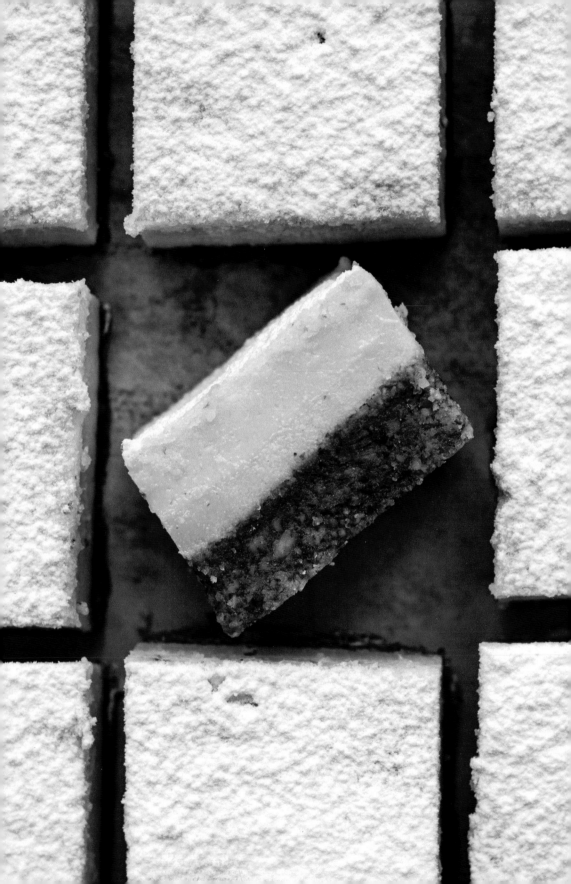

Keto Lemon Bars

Prep Time: 10 minutes | Cook Time: 40 minutes | Total Time: 50 minutes

12 Servings
GF-K-VG

Ingredients For the crust:

- 2 cups almond flour
- 1/2 cup unsalted butter, melted
- 1/3 cup erythritol

Ingredients For the FILLING:

- 5 large eggs
- 1/3 cup lemon juice
- 1/2 cup erythritol
- 2 tbsp coconut flour
- 1/4 cup unsalted butter, melted

Method

1. Preheat the oven to 350°F and line a square 8" pan with parchment paper.
2. In a medium-size bowl, combine the melted butter, powdered sugar and almond flour. It should look like wet sand. Transfer the mixture to your pan and press firmly.
3. Bake the crust for 13-15 minutes or until slightly golden. While your crust is in the oven, prepare your filling.
4. In a separate mixing bowl, mix your lemon juice, melted butter and sweetener. Once the mixture is smooth, add eggs, coconut flour and mix well.
5. Remove the crust from the oven and quickly add the lemon filling.
6. Bake for 22-25 minutes or until the center is slightly jiggly.
7. Remove the cake from the oven and let it cool down completely before removing it from the pan.
8. Once it is cool and ready to serve, sprinkle some extra sweetener on top.

NUTRITION FACTS

SERVINGS: 4

amount per serving			DV%			DV%
CALORIES **245**	Total Fat	22.4 g	29%	Total Carbohydrates	24.5 g	9%
	Saturated Fat	8.6 g	43%	Dietary Fiber	2 g	7%
NET CARBS **22.5 g**	Cholesterol	108 mg	36%	Total Sugars	20.7 g	
	Sodium	118 mg	5%	Protein	6.8 g	

Appendix

Appendix A: Get Moving

Appendix B: Sugar Related Diseases

Appendix C: No Sugar Co. Products

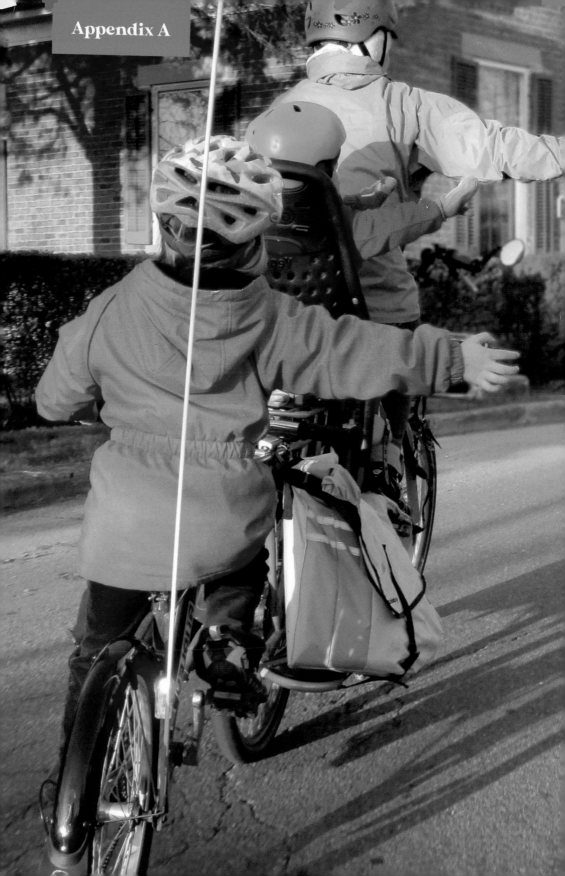

GET MOVING!

A big part of the No Sugar In Me life-style is being active. While we touched on it earlier in the book, it's important to look at your activity level as part of the lifestyle that comes with the improvements outlined in this book. However, before you decide to devote yourself to activities that may be beyond your current capabilities, you need to know that what you do to stay active each day is less important than how you do it.

Any physical activity that gets your heart rate going can fit in this life-style. But any expert in the health and fitness industry will tell you that there are methods to achieving optimal results. In all the years I've worked around fitness professionals, the best advice I've seen consistently over the duration of my career is that if you want to lose weight, promote lean muscle gains, and simply get healthier, your best bet is to approach physical activity with intervals. While it may sound complicated to someone who hasn't ever done them, inter-val training is actually quite simple. Here's a sample interval workout that can apply to any physical activity for someone at any fitness level:

Warm up: 30 seconds at a slow pace
Round 1: 30 seconds half speed, 30 seconds slow pace, 30 seconds all-out sprint, 30 seconds slow pace.

Repeat five times for 10 minutes or jump into round 2 for an intermedi-ate level.
Round 2: 1 minute half speed, 15 seconds slow pace, 1 minute all-out sprint, 15 seconds slow pace. Repeat 4 times for a 10 minute, intense quick workout or jump back to round 1 to wind down and finish. Or, if you want something advanced, move on to round 3.
Round 3: 15 seconds half speed, 90 seconds all out sprint, 15 seconds half speed, 2 minutes all out sprint Repeat three times and then do round 2 and finish with round 1.

This simple workout relies on you being the judge of your own exertion and allows you to decide what you can do and for how long you should do it. The best part is that you can apply this interval workout to virtually any physical activity! No matter what you decide, if you follow this ap-proach, you'll see yourself benefiting from every minute you're being active. For beginners, keep moving your body in a way that feels comfortable and challenge yourself a bit further every day. You can even start with just one minute a day with something as sim-ple as a stretch, and then add another minute the next day. Work your way up to 30 minutes and your body will thank you. So, go ahead!

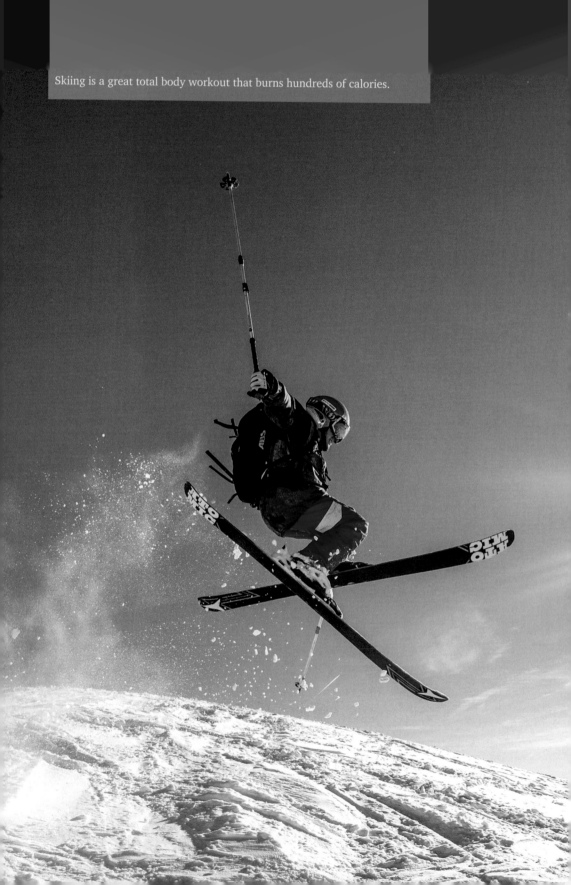

Skiing is a great total body workout that burns hundreds of calories.

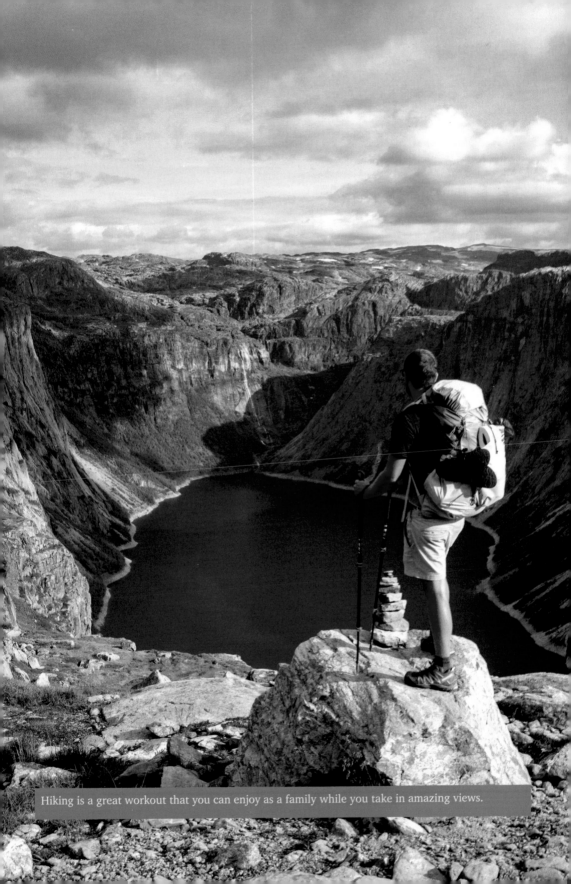

Hiking is a great workout that you can enjoy as a family while you take in amazing views.

Sugar Related Diseases

Clinical research that is linking sugar to a number of serious conditions is growing worldwide. Study by study, they are pointing to sugar as the culprit for eroding our health. It may take years for regulating bodies and governments to step in and get involved the way they did with other substances like drugs and tobacco. Until then, it is up to us to be aware of the potential dangers and try our best to protect ourselves. I intentionally didn't want to include every health condition that sugar has been linked to as that would have made for a very lengthy book. Instead, I am including some of the highlights of the research that I have come across over the years in this Appendix along with references, should you like to learn more.

Addiction and Sugar

Is sugar addictive and why do we like it so much? Addiction is a very strong word that evokes an emotional reaction so I will say that sugar as an addiction is a heavily debated topic. From an evolutionary perspective, it makes complete sense as to why we enjoy eating sweet foods.

Going back to the days of hunter and gatherer societies, finding a sweet food indicated that it was safe to eat and that it contained a high caloric intake. Meaning, that we would satisfy our hunger for longer periods of time. But back in those days, the primary source of sugar came from fruits that were eaten on rare occasions.

From a physiological perspective, small amounts of sugar are useful as an energy source that gets distributed throughout our bodies. Sugar also triggers reward centers in our brains, releasing feel-good chemicals like dopamine, serotonin, and endorphins. These chemicals in turn trigger the feeling of satisfaction.[77] However, that satisfaction is temporary and over time, fades in intensity.

One of the issues with eating sugar is that the more we eat it, the more our taste buds get used to that level of sugar intake and in turn, we crave higher volume to experience that same level of satisfaction. In other words, the more we eat it, the more we crave it. This mechanism loop is exactly what happens with other forms of addiction, where the more you consume, the higher the tolerance that you build is and the higher the quantity you'll need to reach that high again.

Researchers from California, New York and Venezuela recently concluded that the feelings a person gets from a sugar high are identical to what other addicts experience. Beyond merely suggesting that sugar can be addictive, they unequivocally concluded that sugar addiction is very real and quite widespread. Their research indicated that sugar addiction shared several basic criteria defined in the Diagnostic and Statistical Manual of Mental Disorders with other forms of substance abuse disorders.[78] The five overlapping criteria include:

- Use of larger amounts and for longer than intended
- Cravings
- Hazardous use
- Increasing tolerance
- Withdrawal

Sugar behaves like a drug in our systems, causing rushes, crashes, and intense cravings as it is an appetite stimulant. Over time, increasing intake of refined sugar not only changes our preferences and taste buds, but is also likely to lead to consumption of higher volume of calories, excess weight and in some cases, eating disorders.[79] While the ongoing debate of whether excessive sugar consumption should be classified as a form of addiction or not continues, it is certainly something for us as a general public to be aware of.

Autoimmune Diseases

Autoimmune diseases occur when antibodies that are supposed to be fighting foreign bodies such as bacteria and viruses attack our own bodies instead, causing severe damage. Many conditions fall into this category, a few of which include Rheumatoid Arthritis, Crohn's Disease, Multiple Sclerosis, Psoriasis, Lupus and Graves' Disease. All of these are serious conditions that are very often a lifelong battle and difficult to treat.

Research published in the Immunity Journal created a serious cause for alarm that linked sugar to Crohn's disease, colitis, and autoimmune encephalomyelitis. The study found that a higher level of sugar consumption led to heightened levels of Th17, which is an inflammatory immune cell that plays a significant role in the destruction of healthy tissue in autoimmune diseases.[80] While research in this space is still in its infancy, a 2019 study proved that mice who were given high sugar intake worsened their autoimmune diseases.[81] As such, low-sugar diets are recommended for anyone who suffers from autoimmune disease.

Chronic Inflammation

Inflammation is our body's natural defense against infection, toxins, or injuries. It sends an army of antibodies, proteins, and increased blood flow to the affected area in an effort to heal faster. This is great defense mechanism that typically lasts up to a few days. Chronic inflammation on the other hand is when the inflammation defense response extends over a larger period of time, sometimes years. This naturally puts a strain on our body as it is hard to sustain over long periods of time and can actually cause damage to the healthy organs.

Did you know that people with diets that are high in sugar have more inflammatory markers in their blood? When you eat sugar, the production of free fatty acids in the liver is instigated and when they are digested into the body the inflammatory process is triggered. Some research indicates that the biggest reaction happens when you consume fructose, which is the most common added sugar in most unhealthy diets. The research also indicates that when people make an active choice to reduce sugar in their diet, especially those in sugar-packed drinks, the inflammation factors in their blood are noticeably decreased.[82]

Alzheimer's and Dementia

Sugar also impacts our brain health. When you think of degenerative brain conditions like Alzheimer's Disease or Dementia, you're probably not thinking about sugar, but recent research indicates that there is a link between high sugar levels in our blood and brain's inability to use it normally. It seems that having high blood sugar can increase the risk of developing Alzheimer's Disease as it impairs cognitive function and increases cognitive decline.[83] Recent research also highlighted that people with Type 2 diabetes are at least twice as likely to develop Alzheimer's. Similarly, those with prediabetes have a higher likelihood of predementia or Mild Cognitive Impairment.[84] The one thing that I hope is becoming very apparent is the compounding effect of how all of these conditions link to one another and lead to higher risks of co-morbidities. While more research needs to be done on the subject of refined sugar and brain health specifically, it's clear that a sugar-heavy diet is likely to have a negative effect on our brain function as well.

Liver Disease

The liver is our second largest organ and is somewhat underrated as it performs over 500 different tasks! Its primary role is to keep our body healthy by processing everything that we ingest and figuring out what toxins to push out of the body, and what to keep, store, and distribute. It is such a vital and complex organ that in the case of severe liver damage, the only solution is to have a transplanted liver. Our livers work as a reservoir for the circulation of blood sugar and other elements that fuel our body, keeping them in steady balance. If our bodies are running low on sugar, the liver can also produce alternative fuels or ketones from fats.[85]

When it comes to refined sugar, it seems that high intake of it can be as damaging to our liver as alcohol, even for those who are not overweight.[86]

In the last 40 years, the medical community has been tracking liver conditions that are linked to sugar consumption: Non-alcoholic fatty liver disease (NAFLD) and Non-alcoholic steatohepatitis (NASH). While we won't go into the details behind these, it's important to note that the growth of these conditions also increased as processed sugar became more prevalent in our diets. Six million Americans currently struggle with NASH and more than 30% of the population is dealing with NAFLD.[87]

There are other liver conditions such as chronic kidney disease, fatty liver disease, and sugar belly that are further adding to this complex storyline. One important thing

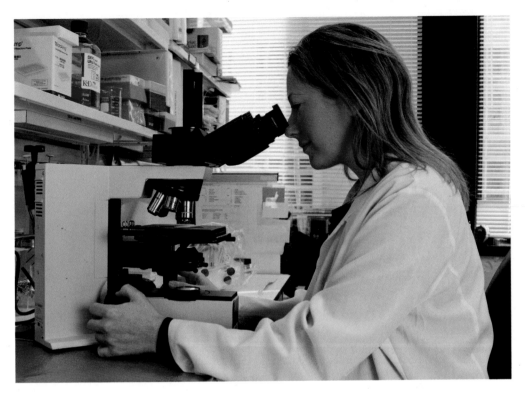

to note is that if your waist is bigger than your hips, you should immediately consult your family doctor, asking for a blood test to check your triglyceride levels and investigate your likelihood of having these liver complications.[88]

While the medical community is still exploring the direct causal relationship between refined sugars and the strain that it puts on our livers, increasing your chances of protecting such a vital organ is yet another reason to limit your sugar intake.

Premature Aging

If all this talk about the chronic conditions hasn't scared you enough to quit sugar, let me also appeal to your vanity. Whether you're young or old, overweight or thin, male or female, refined sugar has a detri-

mental effect on your skin as well. Yes, genetics have a huge impact on how our skin ages but regardless of our genetic makeup, consuming large quantities of sugar can accelerate our aging process. As sugar enters our body and blood stream, it can attach itself to collagen and elastin in skin.[89] When this happens, our skin loses its elasticity, leading to wrinkles and sagging skin.[90]

If that's not bad enough, consumption of refined sugar also leads to inflammation, which can further irritate skin conditions, leading to broken capillaries, acne, or eczema. Lastly, as our bodies acquire a larger caloric intake from refined sugars, it is simultaneously deprived from the good vitamins and minerals in needs for maintenance of healthy, youthful skin.

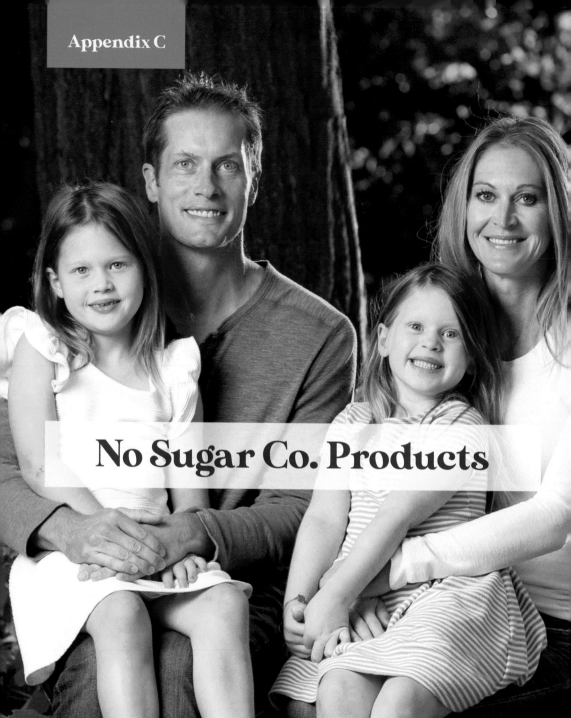

No Sugar Co. Products

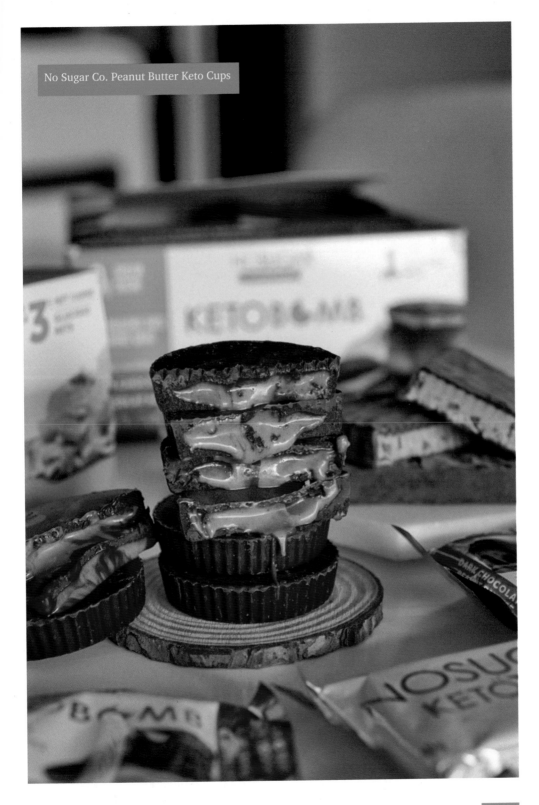

No Sugar Co. Peanut Butter Keto Cups

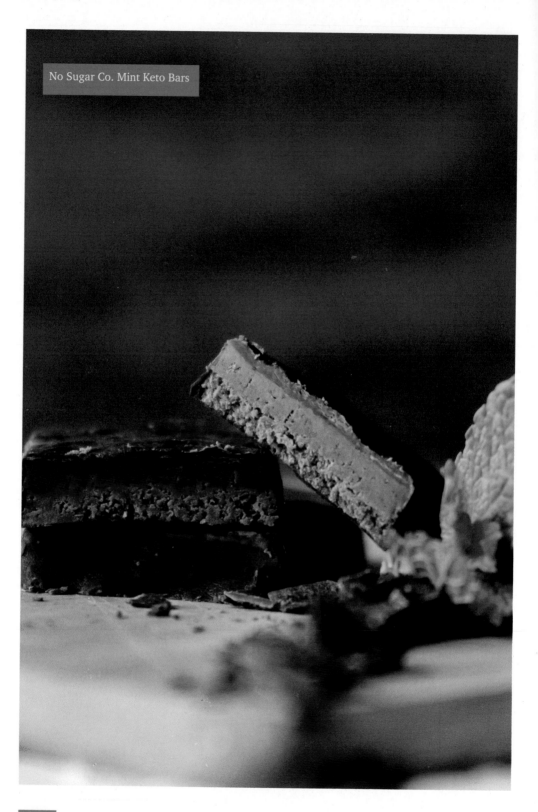

No Sugar Co. Mint Keto Bars

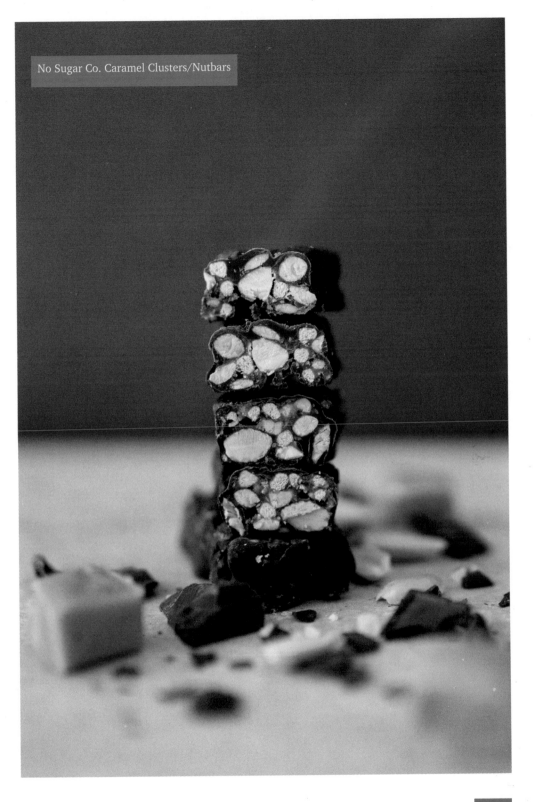

No Sugar Co. Caramel Clusters/Nutbars

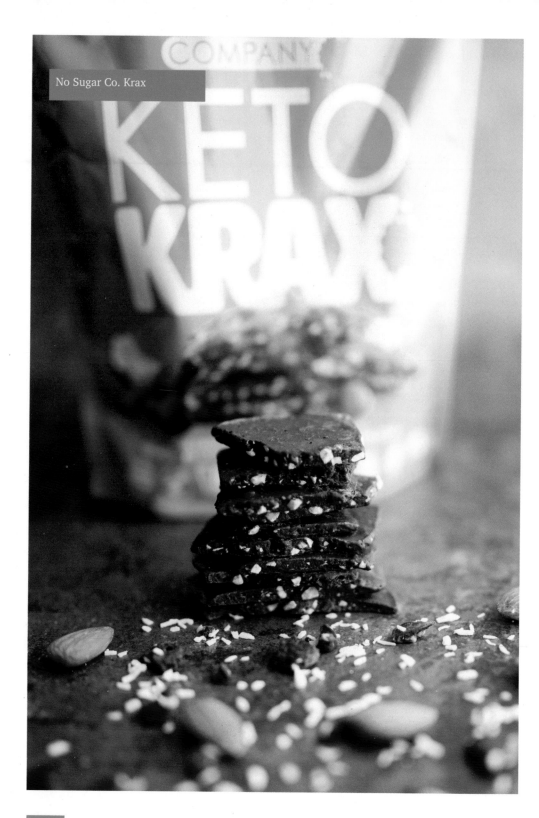

No Sugar Co. Krax

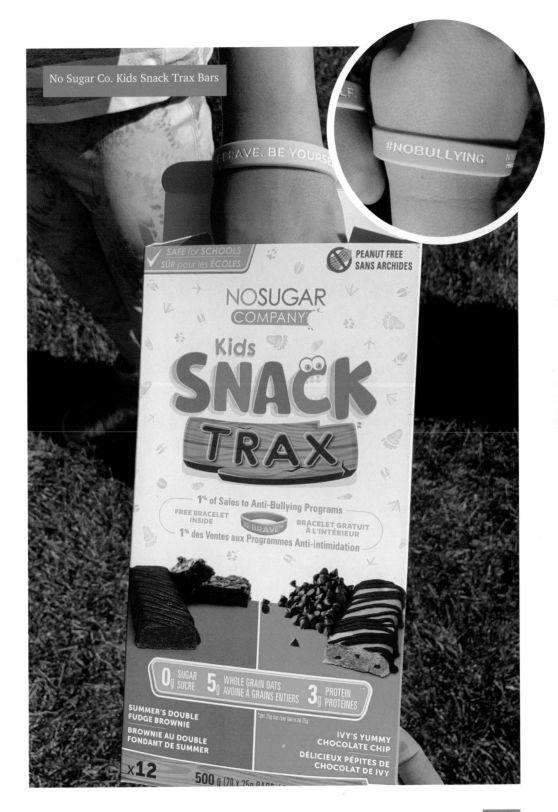

No Sugar Co. Kids Snack Trax Bars

#NOBULLYING

SAFE for SCHOOLS
SÛR pour les ÉCOLES

PEANUT FREE
SANS ARCHIDES

NOSUGAR
COMPANY

Kids
SNACK
TRAX

1% of Sales to Anti-Bullying Programs
FREE BRACELET
INSIDE
BE BRAVE
BRACELET GRATUIT
À L'INTÉRIEUR
1% des Ventes aux Programmes Anti-intimidation

0g SUGAR
SUCRE
5g WHOLE GRAIN OATS
AVOINE À GRAINS ENTIERS
3g PROTEIN
PROTÉINES

SUMMER'S DOUBLE
FUDGE BROWNIE

BROWNIE AU DOUBLE
FONDANT DE SUMMER

IVY'S YUMMY
CHOCOLATE CHIP

DÉLICIEUX PÉPITES DE
CHOCOLAT DE IVY

x12

500 g

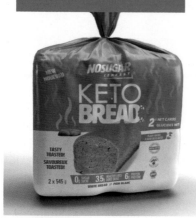

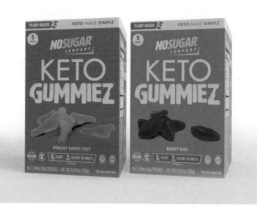

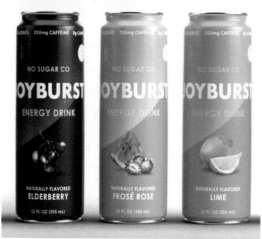

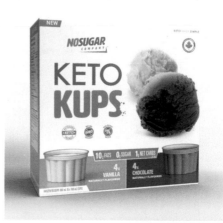

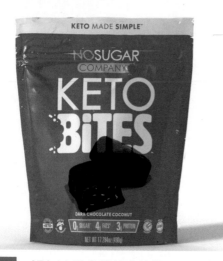

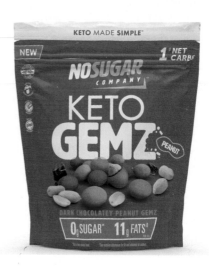

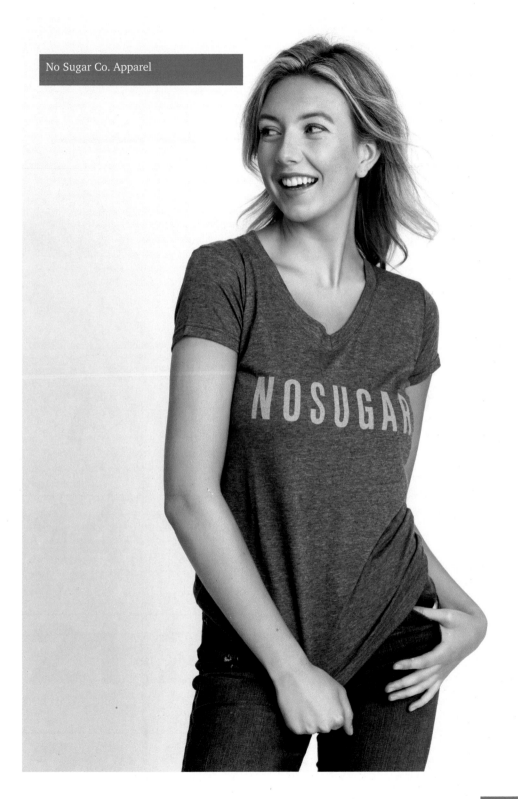

Sources

1   Additional Information about High-Intensity Sweeteners Permitted for Use in Food in the United States. https://www.fda.gov/food/food-additives-petitions/additional-information-about-high-intensity-sweeteners-permitted-use-food-united-states.

2   Fogelholm M, Anderssen S, Gunnarsdottir I, Lahti-Koski M. Dietary macronutrients and food consumption as determinants of long-term weight change in adult populations: a systematic literature review. Food Nutr Res. 2012;56:10.3402/fnr.v56i0.19103. doi:10.3402/fnr.v56i0.19103.

3   How Does Sugar Affect the Skin? October 2019. https://www.biodermis.com/how-does-sugar-affect-the-skin-s/297.htm

4   Mantantzis K, Schlaghecken F, Sünram-Lea SI, Maylor EA. Sugar rush or sugar crash? A meta-analysis of carbohydrate effects on mood. Neurosci Biobehav Rev. 2019 Jun;101:45-67. doi: 10.1016/j.neubiorev.2019.03.016. Epub 2019 Apr 3. PMID: 30951762.

5   Kjeldsen JS, Hjorth MF, Andersen R, Michaelsen KF, Tetens I, Astrup A, Chaput JP, Sjödin A. Short sleep duration and large variability in sleep duration are independently associated with dietary risk factors for obesity in Danish school children. Int J Obes (Lond). 2014 Jan;38(1):32-9. doi: 10.1038/ijo.2013.147. Epub 2013 Aug 8. PMID: 23924757.

6   The alarming truth about how sugar ruins your sleep. https://www.theguardian.com/lifeandstyle/2020/jan/12/the-alarming-truth-about-how-sugar-ruins-your-sleep

7   Ginieis R, Franz EA, Oey I, Peng M. The "sweet" effect: comparative assessments of dietary sugars on cognitive performance. Physiol Behav. 2018;184(December 2017):242–247.

8   The Best and Worst Foods for Your Teeth. https://www.urmc.rochester.edu/encyclopedia/content.aspx?ContentTypeID=1&ContentID=4062

9   Masana MF, Tyrovolas S, Kolia N, et al. Dietary Patterns and Their Association with Anxiety Symptoms among Older Adults: The ATTICA Study. Nutrients. 2019;11(6):1250. Published 2019 May 31. doi:10.3390/nu11061250.

10   Fat Chance: Beating the Odds Against Sugar, Processed Food, Obesity, and Disease; Robert H. Lustig M.D., 2017.

11   Additional Information about High-Intensity Sweeteners Permitted for Use in Food in the United States. https://www.fda.gov/food/food-additives-petitions/additional-information-about-high-intensity-sweeteners-permitted-use-food-united-states

12   Additional Information about High-Intensity Sweeteners Permitted for Use in Food in the United States. https://www.fda.gov/food/food-additives-petitions/additional-information-about-high-intensity-sweeteners-permitted-use-food-united-states

13   Goyal SK, Samsher, Goyal RK. Stevia (Stevia rebaudiana) a bio-sweetener: a review. Int J Food Sci Nutr. 2010 Feb;61(1):1-10. doi: 10.3109/09637480903193049. PMID: 19961353.

14   Natural Food Additives, Ingredients and Flavourings. A volume in Woodhead Publishing Series in Food Science, Technology and Nutrition. Book 2012. David Baines and Richard Seal.

15   Noda K, Nakayama K, Oku T. Serum glucose and insulin levels and erythritol balance after oral administration of erythritol in healthy subjects. Eur J Clin Nutr. 1994 Apr;48(4):286-92. PMID: 8039489.

16   Hidden in Plain Sight--Added sugar is hiding in 74% of packaged foods. https://sugarscience.ucsf.edu/hidden-in-plain-sight/#.YGOp269KhPZ

17   Mucci, Kristy. The Illustrated History of How Sugar Conquered the World. January 9, 2017. https://www.saveur.com/sugar-history-of-the-world/

18   Guideline: sugars intake for adults and children. March 4, 2015. https://www.who.int/publications/i/item/9789241549028

19   Murandu M, Webber MA, Simms MH, Dealey C. Use of granulated sugar therapy in the management of sloughy or necrotic wounds: a pilot study. J Wound Care. 2011 May;20(5):206, 208, 210 passim. doi: 10.12968/jowc.2011.20.5.206. PMID: 21647066.

20   History of Sugar. https://www.sugar.org/sugar/history/

21   Shahbandeh, M. June 3, 2020. Total sugar consumption worldwide from 2009/2010 to 2020/2021 (in million metric tons). https://www.statista.com/statistics/249681/total-consumption-of-sugar-worldwide/

22   Koivistoinen P, Hyvönen L. The use of sugar in foods. Int Dent J. 1985 Sep;35(3):175-9. PMID: 3863796.

23   Wiss David A., Avena Nicole, Rada Pedro. Sugar Addiction: From Evolution to Revolution. Frontiers in Psychiatry, Volume 9, 2018. https://www.frontiersin.org/article/10.3389/fpsyt.2018.00545.

24   Interlandi, Jeneel. April 9, 2020. The U.S. Approach to Public Health: Neglect, Panic, Repeat. https://www.nytimes.com/2020/04/09/opinion/sunday/coronavirus-public-health-system-us.html

25   U.S. Department of Health and Human Services and U.S. Department of Agriculture. 2015 – 2020 Dietary Guidelines for Americans. 8th Edition. December 2015.

26   How much sugar do you eat? You may be surprised. https://www.dhhs.nh.gov/dphs/nhp/documents/sugar.pdf

27   Kearns CE, Schmidt LA, Glantz SA. Sugar Industry and Coronary Heart Disease Research: A Historical Analysis of Internal Industry Documents. JAMA Intern Med. 2016;176(11):1680–1685.

28   How the Sugar Industry Shifted Blame to Fat. https://www.nytimes.com/2016/09/13/well/eat/how-the-sugar-industry-shifted-blame-to-fat.html

29   Domonoske, Camila. September 13, 2016. 50 Years Ago, Sugar Industry Quietly Paid Scientists To Point Blame At Fat. https://www.npr.org/sections/thetwo-way/2016/09/13/493739074/50-years-ago-sugar-industry-quietly-paid-scientists-to-point-blame-at-fat

30   Te Morenga L, Mallard S, Mann J. Dietary sugars and body weight: systematic review and meta-analyses of randomised controlled trials and cohort studies BMJ 2013; 346 :e7492 doi:10.1136/bmj.e7492.

31   Adult Obesity. https://www.hsph.harvard.edu/obesity-prevention-source/obesity-trends/obesity-rates-worldwide/

32   Wei, Yau. October 19, 2020. The Relationship Between Obesity, Diabetes and the Heart. https://www.mountelizabeth.com.sg/healthplus/article/the-relationship-between-obesity-diabetes-and-the-heart

33   Diabetes and Obesity. https://www.diabetes.co.uk/diabetes-and-obesity.html

34   Waters, Hugh. September 22, 2020. America's Obesity Crisis: The Health and Economic Costs of Excess Weight. https://milkeninstitute.org/reports/americas-obesity-crisis-health-and-economic-costs-excess-weight

35   Obesity and overweight. https://www.who.int/news-room/fact-sheets/detail/obesity-and-overweight

36   Stanhope KL. Sugar consumption, metabolic disease and obesity: The state of the controversy. Crit Rev Clin Lab Sci. 2016;53(1):52-67. doi: 10.3109/10408363.2015.1084990. Epub 2015 Sep 17. PMID: 26376619; PMCID: PMC4822166.

37   Rowley WR, Bezold C, Arikan Y, Byrne E, Krohe S. Diabetes 2030: Insights from Yesterday, Today, and Future Trends. Popul Health Manag. 2017;20(1):6-12. doi:10.1089/pop.2015.0181.

38   Diabetes. https://www.hopkinsmedicine.org/endoscopic-weight-loss-program/conditions/diabetes.html

39   The sweet danger of sugar. https://www.health.harvard.edu/heart-health/the-sweet-danger-of-sugar#

40   DiNicolantonio JJ, Lucan SC. The wrong white crystals: not salt but sugar as aetiological in hypertension and cardiometabolic disease. Open Heart 2014;1:e000167. doi: 10.1136/openhrt-2014-000167.

41   Patton, Katherine. June 4, 2018. How Small, Frequent Meals Can Help Athletes Keep Energy High. https://health.clevelandclinic.org/how-small-frequent-meals-can-help-athletes-keep-energy-high/

42   Elliott, Brianna. August 9, 2017. 19 Water-Rich Foods That Help You Stay Hydrated. https://www.healthline.com/nutrition/19-hydrating-foods#

43   Laskowski, Edward. What are the risks of sitting too much? https://www.mayoclinic.org/healthy-lifestyle/adult-health/expert-answers/sitting/faq-20058005

44   Fiorenzi, Ryan. January 31, 2021. Sitting Is The New Smoking. https://www.startstanding.org/sitting-new-smoking/#extended

45   Tal A, Wansink B. Fattening Fasting: Hungry Grocery Shoppers Buy More Calories, Not More Food. JAMA Intern Med. 2013;173(12):1146–1148. doi:10.1001/jamainternmed.2013.650.

46   Baron KG, Reid KJ, Kern AS, Zee PC. Role of sleep timing in caloric intake and BMI. Obesity (Silver Spring). 2011 Jul;19(7):1374-81. doi: 10.1038/oby.2011.100. Epub 2011 Apr 28. PMID: 21527892.

47   Donga E, van Dijk M, van Dijk JG, Biermasz NR, Lammers GJ, van Kralingen KW, Corssmit EP, Romijn JA. A single night of partial sleep deprivation induces insulin resistance in multiple metabolic pathways in healthy subjects. J Clin Endocrinol Metab. 2010 Jun;95(6):2963-8. doi: 10.1210/jc.2009-2430. Epub 2010 Apr 6. PMID: 20371664.

48   Buxton OM, Cain SW, O'Connor SP, Porter JH, Duffy JF, Wang W, Czeisler CA, Shea SA. Adverse metabolic consequences in humans of prolonged sleep restriction combined with circadian disruption. Sci Transl Med. 2012 Apr 11;4(129):129ra43. doi: 10.1126/scitranslmed.3003200. PMID: 22496545; PMCID: PMC3678519.

49   Meng X, Li Y, Li S, et al. Dietary Sources and Bioactivities of Melatonin. Nutrients. 2017;9(4):367. Published 2017 Apr 7. doi:10.3390/nu9040367.

50   Scheer FA, Morris CJ, Shea SA. The internal circadian clock increases hunger and appetite in the evening independent of food intake and other behaviors. Obesity (Silver Spring). 2013;21(3):421-423. doi:10.1002/oby.20351.

51   Gupta, Sanjay. January 2021. Keep Sharp: Build a Better Brain at Any Age. 183-184.

52   Magnesium. https://ods.od.nih.gov/factsheets/Magnesium-HealthProfessional/#h7.

53   Wheless JW. History of the ketogenic diet. Epilepsia. 2008 Nov;49 Suppl 8:3-5. doi: 10.1111/j.1528-1167.2008.01821.x. PMID: 19049574.

54   https://www.forbes.com/sites/jennifercohen/2020/01/23/hottest-diets-of-2020/?sh=2a008e825b35

55   https://www.healthline.com/nutrition/ketogenic-diet-foods

56   https://www.healthline.com/nutrition/15-conditions-benefit-ketogenic-diet

57   https://www.medicalnewstoday.com/articles/320929

58   https://www.everydayhealth.com/diet-nutrition/ketogenic-diet/comprehensive-ketogenic-diet-food-list-follow/

59   https://www.webmd.com/diet/obesity/features/not-all-carbs-are-created-equally#1

60   Ebbeling C B, Feldman H A, Klein G L, Wong J M W, Bielak L, Steltz S K et al. Effects of a low carbohydrate diet on energy expenditure during weight loss maintenance: randomized trial BMJ 2018; 363 :k4583 doi:10.1136/bmj.k4583

61   https://perfectketo.com/how-to-exercise-in-ketosis/

62   https://www.active.com/food-and-nutrition/articles/6-ways-you-can-train-your-brain-to-lose-weight

63   https://www.nature.com/articles/ijo2017206

64   Monica P. McNamara, Jennifer M. Singleton, Marcell D. Cadney, Paul M. Ruegger, James Borneman, Theodore Garland. February 25, 2021. Journal of Experimental Biology 2021 224: jeb239699 doi: 10.1242/jeb.239699.

65   Scientific Report of the 2020 Dietary Guidelines Advisory Committee. July 2020. https://www.dietaryguidelines.gov/sites/default/files/2020-07/ScientificReport_of_the_2020DietaryGuidelinesAdvisoryCommittee_first-print.pdf

66   Healthy Kids are Sweet Enough. https://www.heart.org/en/healthy-living/healthy-eating/eat-smart/sugar/sugar-recommendation-healthy-kids-and-teens-infographic

67   How Much Candy Is Sold on Halloween? March 25, 2020. https://www.reference.com/world-view/much-candy-sold-halloween-ee3f0bd8ac01852

68   Molteni R, Barnard RJ, Ying Z, Roberts CK, Gómez-Pinilla F. A high-fat, refined sugar diet reduces hippocampal brain-derived neurotrophic factor, neuronal plasticity, and learning. Neuroscience. 2002;112(4):803-14. doi: 10.1016/s0306-4522(02)00123-9. PMID: 12088740.

69   What to Do When Your Child Eats Too Much Sugar. March 26, 2020. https://health.clevelandclinic.org/what-to-do-when-your-child-eats-too-much-sugar/

70   Bentley, R. Alexander. U.S. obesity as delayed effect of excess sugar. Economics & Human Biology, Volume 36, 2020. 100818, ISSN 1570-677X. https://doi.org/10.1016/j.ehb.2019.100818.

71   Belluck, Pam. March 17, 2005. Children's Life Expectancy Being Cut Short by Obesity. https://www.nytimes.com/2005/03/17/health/childrens-life-expectancy-being-cut-short-by-obesity.html

72   Gillman, Matthew. Family Dinner and Diet Quality Among Older Children and Adolescents. Arch Fam Med. 2000;9:235-240.

73   Robinson, Eric. Eating attentively: a systematic review and meta-analysis of the effect of food intake memory and awareness on eating, The American Journal of Clinical Nutrition, Volume 97, Issue 4, April 2013, Pages 728–742, https://doi.org/10.3945/ajcn.112.045245.

74   Cooke, L. (2007). The importance of exposure for healthy eating in childhood: a review. Journal of human nutrition and dietetics, 20(4), 294-301.

75   Xiao Z, Lester GE, Luo Y, Wang Q. Assessment of vitamin and carotenoid concentrations of emerging food products: edible microgreens. J Agric Food Chem. 2012 Aug 8;60(31):7644-51. doi: 10.1021/jf300459b. Epub 2012 Jul 30. PMID: 22812633.

76   Buchner, Jill. May 22, 2017. Think giving your kids juice is better than soda? Think again. https://www.todaysparent.com/kids/kids-health/think-giving-your-kids-juice-is-better-than-soda-think-again/

77   Why Is Sugar Addiction A Problem? https://www.addictioncenter.com/drugs/sugar-addiction/

78   Wiss David A., Avena Nicole, Rada Pedro. Sugar Addiction: From Evolution to Revolution. Frontiers in Psychiatry. Volume 9, 2018. https://www.frontiersin.org/article/10.3389/fpsyt.2018.00545. DOI=10.3389/fpsyt.2018.00545.

79   Avena NM, Rada P, Hoebel BG. Evidence for sugar addiction: behavioral and neurochemical effects of intermittent, excessive sugar intake. Neurosci Biobehav Rev. 2008;32(1):20-39. doi:10.1016/j.neubiorev.2007.04.019.

80   Zhang, Dunfang. High Glucose Intake Exacerbates Autoimmunity through Reactive-Oxygen-Species-Mediated TGF- Cytokine Activation. August, 2019. Immunity. https://doi.org/10.1016/j.immuni.2019.08.001.

81   High sugar intake worsens autoimmune disease in mice. August 27, 2019. https://www.nih.gov/news-events/nih-research-matters/high-sugar-intake-worsens-autoimmune-disease-mice

82   Della Corte KW, Perrar I, Penczynski KJ, Schwingshackl L, Herder C, Buyken AE. Effect of Dietary Sugar Intake on Biomarkers of Subclinical Inflammation: A Systematic Review and Meta-Analysis of Intervention Studies. Nutrients. 2018;10(5):606. Published 2018 May 12. doi:10.3390/nu10050606.

83   Gupta, Sanjay MD. Keep Sharp: Build a Better Brain at Any Age. January 2021; 58-60.

84   H.J.Lee, H.I.Seo, H.Y.Cha, et al., Diabetes and Alzheimer's Disease: Mechanisms and Nutritional Aspects. Clinical Nutrition Research 7, no4. (October 2018); 229-240.

85   Digestive Health. What Does the Liver Do, and How Do I Keep Mine Healthy? Rene Wisely November 06, 2017.

86   Abundance of fructose not good for the liver or heart. https://www.health.harvard.edu/heart-health/abundance-of-fructose-not-good-for-the-liver-heart.

87   Browning, Jeffrey. Prevalence of hepatic steatosis in an urban population in the United States: Impact of ethnicity. https://aasldpubs.onlinelibrary.wiley.com/doi/full/10.1002/hep.20466.

88   Kavanagh, Ann. Sugar's Sick Secrets. https://www.ucsf.edu/magazine/sugars-sick-secrets.

89   Danby FW. Nutrition and aging skin: sugar and glycation. Clin Dermatol. 2010 Jul-Aug;28(4):409-11. doi: 10.1016/j.clindermatol.2010.03.018. PMID: 20620757.

90   Nguyen HP, Katta R. Sugar Sag: Glycation and the Role of Diet in Aging Skin. Skin Therapy Lett. 2015 Nov;20(6):1-5. PMID: 27224842.